Brittle Bone Disease Demystified: Doctor's Secret Guide

Dr. Ankita Kashyap and Prof. Krishna N. Sharma

Published by Virtued Press, 2023.

While every precaution has been taken in the preparation of this book, the publisher assumes no responsibility for errors or omissions, or for damages resulting from the use of the information contained herein.

BRITTLE BONE DISEASE DEMYSTIFIED: DOCTOR'S SECRET GUIDE

First edition. October 13, 2023.

Copyright © 2023 Dr. Ankita Kashyap and Prof. Krishna N. Sharma.

ISBN: 979-8223834946

Written by Dr. Ankita Kashyap and Prof. Krishna N. Sharma.

Table of Contents

- 1
- Chapter 1: Understanding Brittle Bone Disease 2
- The Genetics of Brittle Bone Disease 3
- Recognizing the Signs and Symptoms 6
- Different Types of Brittle Bone Disease 8
- Psychological Impact of Brittle Bone Disease 11
- Current Treatment Options 14
- Chapter 2: Holistic Approach to Preventing Brittle Bone Disease 18
- Building Strong Bones Through Nutrition 19
- Exercise and Physical Activity for Bone Strength 22
- Environmental Factors and Bone Health 25
- Lifestyle Modifications for Stronger Bones 28
- Preventive Measures for Brittle Bone Disease 31
- Chapter 3: Managing Brittle Bone Disease 35
- Fracture Prevention and First Aid 36
- Assistive Devices and Adaptive Equipment 39
- Pain Management Strategies 43
- Psychological Support and Coping Strategies 46
- Enhancing Quality of Life 49
- Chapter 4: Complementary and Alternative Therapies 52
- Acupuncture and Traditional Chinese Medicine 53
- Herbal Remedies and Supplements 56
- Mind-Body Practices for Pain Management 59
- Energy Healing Modalities 62
- Integrating Complementary Therapies 65
- Chapter 5: Nurturing Emotional Well-being 68
- Embracing Self-Acceptance and Body Positivity 69
- Overcoming Emotional Challenges 72
- Building Resilience and Mental Strength 74
- Seeking Professional Help 78

Cultivating Supportive Relationships 81
Chapter 6: Empowering Independence and Accessibility 84
Home Modifications for Accessibility 85
Assistive Technology for Independence 88
Accessible Transportation Options 91
Education and Employment Accommodations........................... 94
Promoting Inclusion and Accessibility in Society 97
Chapter 7: Living a Fulfilling Life With Brittle Bone Disease .. 100
Pursuing Personal Goals and Dreams 101
Exploring Adaptive Hobbies and Recreation 104
Advocacy and Making a Difference 108
Celebrating Achievements and Milestones................................. 110
Embracing Positivity and Gratitude 113
Chapter 8: Insights From Brittle Bone Disease Patients 116
Stories of Resilience and Overcoming Challenges 117
Perspectives on Living With Brittle Bone Disease 120
Building Support Networks and Community 123
Promoting Awareness and Advocacy... 126
Lessons Learned and Words of Wisdom 129
Chapter 9: Supporting Friends and Family................................. 133
Educating Yourself About Brittle Bone Disease 134
Communication and Active Listening.. 137
Providing Emotional Support... 140
Practical Assistance and Accommodations 144
Fostering Inclusivity and Advocacy 147
Chapter 10: Research and Advances in Brittle Bone Disease 150
Current Research Studies and Clinical Trials............................. 151
Genetic Discoveries and Therapeutic Targets 154
Regenerative Medicine and Bone Repair 157
Assistive Technologies and Accessibility Innovations 160
Future Directions and Hope... 163
Chapter 11: Building a Supportive Healthcare Team................. 166
Identifying the Right Healthcare Professionals 167

Effective Communication With Healthcare Providers 171
Collaborative Care and Treatment Planning................................ 175
Advocating for Comprehensive Care.. 179
Navigating the Healthcare System 182
Chapter 12: Empowering the Brittle Bone Disease Community... 185
Creating Supportive Networks and Organizations..................... 186
Raising Awareness and Challenging Stigma 190
Sharing Resources and Information 192
Supporting Research and Fundraising... 195
Inspiring Hope and Celebrating Strength..................................... 198

DISCLAIMER

The information provided in this book is intended for general informational purposes only. The content is not meant to substitute professional medical advice, diagnosis, or treatment. Always consult with a qualified healthcare provider before making any changes to your diabetes management plan or healthcare regimen.

While every effort has been made to ensure the accuracy and completeness of the information presented, the author and publisher do not assume any responsibility for errors, omissions, or potential misinterpretations of the content. Individual responses to diabetes management strategies may vary, and what works for one person might not be suitable for another.

The book does not endorse any specific medical treatments, products, or services. Readers are encouraged to seek guidance from their healthcare providers to determine the most appropriate approaches for their unique medical conditions and needs.

Any external links or resources provided in the book are for convenience and informational purposes only. The author and publisher do not have control over the content or availability of these external sources and do not endorse or guarantee the accuracy of such information.

Readers are advised to exercise caution and use their judgment when applying the information provided in this book to their own situations. The author and publisher disclaim any liability for any direct, indirect, consequential, or other damages arising from the use of this book and its content.

By reading and using this book, readers acknowledge and accept the limitations and inherent risks associated with implementing the strategies, recommendations, and information contained herein. It is always recommended to consult a qualified healthcare professional for personalized medical advice and care.

Chapter 1: Understanding Brittle Bone Disease

The Genetics of Brittle Bone Disease

Understanding the genetic basis of brittle bone disease requires a basic understanding of how genes and inheritance work. Our genes, which are the building blocks of heredity, define our characteristics and traits. They are made of DNA molecules and are located on chromosomes in the cell nucleus.

Osteogenesis imperfecta, also referred to as brittle bone disease, is a hereditary disorder that impairs the synthesis of collagen, a protein that provides our bones their strength and shape. The COL1A1 and COL1A2 genes are crucial in the production of collagen.

Most cases of brittle bone disease are caused by mutations in the COL1A1 or COL1A2 genes. The synthesis or structure of collagen may be impacted by certain mutations, which could lead to weak, brittle bones. In some cases, the changes might result in collagen that is more fragile and prone to breaking.

The specific mutation in question may have a varied impact on the brittle bone disease inheritance patterns. Usually, the disease is passed down through an autosomal dominant gene. This indicates that a person only needs to inherit one copy of the defective gene from either parent in order to develop the disease.

However, there have been isolated cases of autosomal recessive inheritance of brittle bone disease. This means that a person must inherit two copies of the damaged gene, one from each parent, in order to have the disorder. In these cases, both parents are typically mutant gene carriers who are unaffected by the disease.

Additionally, occurrences of Brittle Bone Disease could possibly be caused by spontaneous mutations. These mutations appear for the first time in an individual and are not inherited from either parent. Spontaneous mutations can happen during the formation of reproductive cells or in the early stages of embryonic development.

Genetic testing can be used to detect Brittle Bone Disease and can also help identify the exact mutation that is to fault. This can help in figuring out the inheritance pattern and in providing genetic counselling to those who are afflicted and their families. This information can also be used to estimate the likelihood of passing the illness on to future generations.

Researchers have found a number of other genes that, in addition to COL1A1 and COL1A2, may have a role in the development of Brittle Bone Disease. Numerous functions of these genes are involved in the processing of collagen and bone formation.

CRTAP is one such gene that results in a protein necessary for the folding and processing of collagen. Mutations in the CRTAP gene have been associated with Osteogenesis Imperfecta Type VII, a kind of brittle bone disease.

Another gene connected to brittle bone disease is the P3H1 gene, which influences how collagen is changed. Mutations in the P3H1 gene can result in osteogenesis imperfecta type VIII, a severe variation of the disease.

Additionally, research has suggested that gene variations that alter collagen synthesis and production may result in less severe forms of brittle bone disease. These include the SERPINF1 gene, which codes for the PEDF protein, and the IFITM5 gene, which is implicated in bone mineralization.

Understanding the role of these genes in brittle bone disease is crucial for the development of specialised medications and treatments. The disease is now being treated with a focus on preventing fractures, managing pain, and improving overall bone health.

As a proponent of holistic medicine, I am in favour of a full approach to the treatment of Brittle Bone Disease. Changes in lifestyle and self-care practises can dramatically improve the quality of life for persons who have the condition in addition to conventional medical therapy.

A healthy diet is essential for the upkeep of strong bones and the production of collagen. A diet rich in calcium, vitamin D, and other minerals essential for bone health can help to strengthen the bones and prevent fractures. Regular exercise that is tailored to the individual's abilities can aid in boosting overall strength and bone density.

For patients with Brittle Bone Disease, counselling and psychological support can be very beneficial. On an emotional and bodily level, the disease typically causes unique difficulties. By treating the psychological impacts of the disease, people can develop coping mechanisms and enhance their general wellbeing.

In conclusion, brittle bone disease has a wide variety of complex genetic components. Several genes, including COL1A1, COL1A2, CRTAP, P3H1, SERPINF1, and IFITM5, have an impact on the condition. The diagnosis of diseases, genetic counselling, and the creation of specialised treatments can all benefit from an understanding of the inheritance patterns and the functions of specific genes. Additionally, a comprehensive approach that includes lifestyle modifications, self-care techniques, and psychological support is necessary for managing Brittle Bone Disease and improving the standard of living for those who are affected by it...

Recognizing the Signs and Symptoms

There are numerous physical symptoms associated with brittle bone disease, and they might vary from person to person. There are a few common signs and symptoms, nevertheless, that we ought to be aware of. One of the most evident symptoms of brittle bone disease is a propensity for fractures. Contrary to healthy bones, which are able to withstand stress and maintain their structure, bones affected by this disorder are very fragile. Even a slight injury or trauma might result in a fracture. These fractures may appear out of nowhere or may be triggered by seemingly harmless motions. The most important thing to keep in mind is that persons with brittle bone disease can break any bone, not just the typical ones like the arms or legs. They can affect any bone in the body, including the spine, ribs, and even the skull.

Bone anomalies are another red flag to watch out for. The poorer structure of the bones in people with brittle bone disease can cause a number of problems. For instance, bending of the legs is a condition where the legs bow outward due to repeated fractures and healing processes. Patients could also be short or regularly have dental problems. Understanding these physical symptoms will enable us to detect Brittle Bone Disease more rapidly.

It's also crucial to understand the challenges caused by brittle bone disease. One such issue is the start of scoliosis. The term "scoliosis" refers to an unnatural lateral curvature of the spine that can be caused by many fractures and brittle bones. This sickness may cause discomfort, misery, and difficulties with daily tasks. Because it allows for correct care and the potential avoidance of subsequent problems, early identification of scoliosis is crucial.

Another problem to be aware of is hearing loss. According to study, the effects of brittle bone disease on the middle ear's bones may cause hearing loss in patients. The ear's delicate structures can become damaged, which can lead to hearing issues. The auditory health of patients with Brittle Bone Disease should be regularly examined in order to manage any potential hearing damage.

Additionally, breathing problems could be a complication of brittle bone disease. The supporting bones of the ribcage may deteriorate, making it harder for the lungs to expand fully. This could result in difficulty breathing, a reduction in oxygen intake, and a higher risk of respiratory infections. It is essential to recognise these respiratory symptoms in order to attain the highest potential lung function.

In addition to its physical symptoms, Brittle Bone Disease may also have psychological and emotional repercussions on individuals, which must be taken into consideration. The psychological health of patients must be addressed because it can be emotionally difficult to manage a chronic condition like this. Psychology and counselling techniques can be quite beneficial in managing the tension and concern that will unavoidably arise. The assistance of loved ones, close friends, and medical experts can have a significant impact on the general wellness of those with brittle bone disease.

In conclusion, recognising the brittle bone disease warning signs and symptoms is essential for ensuring its early detection and effective treatment. From frequent fractures and bone deformities to repercussions like scoliosis and hearing loss, being aware of these manifestations enables us to provide patients with the support and solutions they need. By implementing a holistic plan that considers their physical, psychological, and emotional requirements, we can improve the quality of life for persons with brittle bone disease and give them the resources they require to live fulfilling lives...

Different Types of Brittle Bone Disease

Type I Brittle Bone Disease:

Type I Brittle Bone Disease, also referred to as Osteogenesis Imperfecta, is the disease's mildest variant. Its defining characteristic is fragile, easily broken bones, especially in childhood and adolescence. One of the primary characteristics that differentiate Type I from other kinds is the propensity for fractures to occur with little to no trauma, or even spontaneously.

Hearing loss, brittle teeth, and blue or grey sclerae are common symptoms in people with Type I brittle bone disease. While some people only fracture once or twice in their lives, others may fracture frequently and find it difficult to go about their daily lives. The degree of the issue can vary significantly.

The major objectives of treatment for Type I brittle bone disease are fracture prevention and the management of related issues. This necessitates a multidisciplinary approach combining orthopaedic surgeons, occupational therapists, and physiotherapists. Patients may use braces or wheelchairs as mobility aids, have surgery to correct skeletal deformities, and arrange routine physiotherapy appointments to strengthen their muscles and improve mobility.

Type II Brittle Bone Disease:

Type II Brittle Bone Disease is the most severe form of the condition. It is characterised by extremely fragile bones, which are frequently present even before birth. Babies born with Type II Brittle Bone Condition usually have an extremely low mortality rate due to the severity of the disease and its associated complications.

Type II is characterised by severe bone abnormalities, frequent short stature, and multiple fractures both during pregnancy and at birth. Additionally, these persons might have breathing problems and skeletal abnormalities that generally reduce their quality of life.

Treatment for Type II Brittle Bone Disease focuses on supportive care in order to maximise patient comfort. Palliative care is typically the mainstay of treatment because of the poor survival rates. For families grieving the tragic loss of a newborn, this involves offering breathing support, emotional support, and pain management.

Type III Brittle Bone Disease:

The severity of Type III brittle bone disease is in the midway of Type I and Type II. People with Type III frequently fracture, especially as children, due to their moderate to severe bone fragility. Unlike Type II Brittle Bone Disease, Type III Brittle Bone Disease fractures frequently occur after birth.

In addition to the disease's characteristic fragile bones, people with Type III brittle bone disease usually have short stature, a barrel-shaped ribcage, and spine curvature. These symptoms may have a significant impact on mobility, necessitating ongoing medical care.

Like Type I brittle bone disease, Type III is managed by preventing fractures and addressing any related issues. Regular physical treatment is necessary to maintain muscular strength and improve mobility. Orthopedic operations could also be necessary to improve bone stability and correct skeletal abnormalities.

Type IV Brittle Bone Disease:

Type IV brittle bone disease is the most complex and changeable type. Its significant bone fragility and high frequency of fractures after delivery make it similar to Type III. Even while Type IV brittle bone disease patients may experience fewer fractures than Type III patients do, the fragility of their bones still causes them considerable complications.

Symptoms of Type IV brittle bone disease are similar to those of other types and include short stature, spine curvature, and skeletal abnormalities. The severity of these symptoms might, however, vary greatly from person to person.

Type IV brittle bone disease is treated in a manner similar to Type I and Type III by reducing the risk of fractures and improving overall quality of life. Regular physical therapy, mobility aids, and orthopaedic operations may be necessary to minimise the condition's impact on daily activities...

Conclusion:

Understanding the many forms of brittle bone disease is essential for providing the best care and assistance to individuals who suffer from it. Each type has unique problems that require specialised treatment methods.

Fractures can result from modest stress in Type I, the least severe form of brittle bone disease. While Type III is of a more moderate severity, Type II is the most dangerous and frequently fatal. The degree of the significant bone fragility linked to Type IV might vary substantially.

By being aware of the ranges in severity, symptoms, and available treatments for Brittle Bone Disease, healthcare professionals may provide tailored care and support to patients. By taking a multidisciplinary approach, placing a focus on preventing fractures, and managing related issues, we can help these people live more fulfilling lives.

Psychological Impact of Brittle Bone Disease

Having brittle bone disease can be emotionally stressful in many ways. First and foremost, persistent worry about fractures and injuries can have a negative impact on a person's mental health. Imagine going about your everyday activities while being aware that a simple fall or even a small bump could result in a fracture. The immense fear and anxiety that accompany this understanding may lead to a chronic state of hypervigilance and worry.

People with brittle bone disease may experience significant effects on their emotional health due to their pain and physical limitations. The illness can cause recurring fractures and persistent pain, which can lead to feelings of frustration, helplessness, and even despair. Simple tasks like standing or walking might become difficult for these people on a regular basis, which further decreases their self-esteem and has a detrimental effect on their general mental health.

Patients with brittle bone disease, their families, and those people in close proximity to them are all affected. Family members frequently go through a variety of other feelings, such as regret, anxiety, and a constant sense of responsibility for the safety of a loved one. In particular, parents could feel constant anxiety from trying to protect their children from harm. Living in a constant state of anxiety may be incredibly tiring and leave little time for self-care and wellbeing maintenance.

Along with emotional challenges, those who have brittle bone disease may also struggle with mental health issues. Feelings of isolation and loneliness might be brought on by physical limitations and continuous suffering. Many patients may experience difficulties accepting themselves and having positive self-images as a result of their physical deformities and frequent fractures. As a result, it may be challenging to forge and maintain bonds while also contributing to social anxiety.

Additionally, the long-term consequences of brittle bone disease, such as movement restrictions and dependency on others for daily activities, can evoke feelings of loss and grief. Accepting the limitations brought on by the illness and finding a new normal can be a difficult and ongoing journey for patients and their families.

But it's important to keep in mind that those who have brittle bone disease are incredibly resilient. Despite the challenges they face, many people are able to control the disease's psychological impacts and enjoy fulfilling lives. The following coping strategies have proven to be helpful for my patients:

1. Seeking support: It can be quite beneficial to advise patients and their families to ask for aid from those who have experienced similar situations. Members of support groups experience a sense of acceptance, understanding, and affirmation. Making connections with individuals who actually comprehend what they are going through lessens emotions of loneliness and offers practical advice for battling day-to-day challenges.

2. Practicing self-care: Patients with Brittle Bone Disease must prioritise taking care of themselves. This can include engaging in hobbies, learning relaxation techniques, or engaging in light exercise regimens—activities that lower stress and improve wellness in general. Participating in rewarding hobbies can considerably improve mental health.

3. Seeking professional help: Those who are struggling with depression, anxiety, or other mental health concerns must get professional help immediately. With the aid of therapists and counsellors who specialise in chronic disease and disability, Brittle Bone Disease's emotional challenges can be managed.

4. Developing resilience: Building resilience is essential for healing any chronic illness' psychological side effects. Patients with brittle bone

disease may find it easier to handle the challenges and uncertainties of living with the condition if they are encouraged to focus on their strengths, set realistic goals, and maintain a positive outlook.

5. Educating oneself and loved ones: knowledge's influence. By being informed about the ailment, its symptoms, and the available therapies, people and their families can make informed decisions and feel more in charge of their situations. Knowledge of the most recent advancements and research in the area of brittle bone disease is essential.

As a practitioner of holistic medicine, I firmly believe that it is important to address both the psychological consequences of a disease and its outward symptoms. By recognising and addressing the emotional challenges, mental health problems, and coping methods for patients with Brittle Bone Disease, we may provide holistic care that promotes overall wellbeing.

In conclusion, persons with brittle bone disease experience severe psychological repercussions in addition to physical challenges. Physical constraints, persistent pain, and fear of fractures can all have a negative impact on mental health. However, if they receive the right care, coping skills, and attention to holistic healthcare, people with brittle bone disease can live happy lives. I believe this chapter has provided clear explanations of the psychological impacts of brittle bone disease and practical advice for addressing and resolving these challenges...

Current Treatment Options

The best way to treat brittle bone disease varies from person to person. Because each patient is unique, their care needs to be tailored to meet their specific needs. As a doctor who promotes holistic healthcare and wellness, I believe in taking a comprehensive approach that addresses both the physical and emotional components of the problem.

Medical Interventions:

Medical interventions are crucial for managing Brittle Bone Disease. Among the medications that are most frequently given to patients with this condition are bisphosphonates. By reducing bone resorption, these drugs lower the risk of fractures. They are frequently administered intravenously or orally to ensure their efficacy and minimise side effects.

In addition to bisphosphonates, other medications can be used to treat the signs and symptoms of brittle bone disease, such as calcitonin and teriparatide. Calcitonin, a hormone, helps regulate the body's calcium and phosphate levels, and teriparatide, a synthetic parathyroid hormone, encourages bone formation. These medications can help increase bone density and reduce the risk of fractures.

Surgical Procedures:

Patients with severe forms of brittle bone disease or those who fracture frequently may need surgical interventions. By executing a series of surgical procedures to stabilise and strengthen the bones, the risk of fractures can be reduced.

An ordinary surgical procedure involves placing metal rods or plates inside the bones. These devices work as internal stabilising supports that assist prevent further fractures. With extreme care, the titanium or stainless steel rods or plates are inserted into the shattered bones and secured. This surgery allows patients to live more active lives by significantly increasing bone strength and mobility.

In some cases, bone grafting may be required to repair and replace damaged bone tissue. In order to treat the injury, healthy bone tissue must be taken from another part of the patient's body or from a donor and transplanted there. This increases the bones' overall toughness and longevity and promotes the growth of new bone...

Supportive Therapies:

Supportive therapies significantly improve the quality of life for individuals with Brittle Bone Disease, even if surgical procedures and pharmaceutical treatments are crucial for controlling the condition. By addressing the physical, emotional, and psychological aspects of the condition, these treatments aim to provide comprehensive therapy.

Physical therapy is a vital form of supportive therapy for people with Brittle Bone Disease. To improve the patient's balance, flexibility, and muscle strength, a competent physiotherapist works closely with the patient to design a personalised exercise programme. These exercises are designed to promote mobility and lower the risk of fractures, enabling patients to go about their daily lives with greater assurance and comfort.

Occupational therapy, which tries to maintain patients' independence and help them adapt to their daily routines, is another form of supportive therapy. Patients and occupational therapists work together to develop safer methods for eating, bathing, and clothing. They may offer aids like adaptable equipment or adapted utensils to make these tasks easier and reduce the chance of damage.

Since Brittle Bone Disease frequently has a negative effect on its patients' emotional health, patients with the condition must also get psychiatric care. Due to managing recurring fractures, chronic pain, and physical limitations, patients may feel frustrated, anxious, or depressed. As a result, counselling and therapy sessions are an essential part of the whole therapeutic approach.

During counselling sessions, patients can express their concerns, thoughts, and feelings concerning their disease in a safe setting.

Patients can benefit from the support of a skilled counsellor or psychologist in developing resiliency, coping strategies, and a positive outlook to help them cope with the challenges of having Brittle Bone Disease. They may also involve family members or caregivers in the therapeutic process to ensure that the patient has a strong support system.

In addition to these supportive therapies, patients with Brittle Bone Disease may also benefit from incorporating complementary and alternative medical practises into their treatment plan. People have found that practises like acupuncture, yoga, and meditation help them relax, release tension, and feel better all around. Even though they might not directly affect bone density or fracture prevention, these techniques can complement traditional medical interventions and supportive therapies by encouraging a holistic feeling of wellness...

Conclusion:

Brittle bone disease can be treated in a variety of ways, but doing so requires a comprehensive plan that considers both the physical and emotional aspects of the condition. For symptom management and fracture prevention, medical interventions such teriparatide, calcitonin, and bisphosphonates are crucial. Examples of surgical procedures that can strengthen the bones and increase mobility include the implantation of rods or plates and bone grafting.

Supportive therapies like physical therapy, occupational therapy, and counselling are crucial for improving the quality of life for people with Brittle Bone Disease. In order for patients to have more fulfilling lives, these treatments place a strong emphasis on patients' emotional health, flexibility, and physical strength. To promote holistic wellness, complementary and alternative medical practises might be integrated.

As a physician and health and wellness coach, I encourage a thorough and personalised therapy strategy that considers each patient's unique requirements and circumstances. By combining medication, surgery, supportive therapy, and complementary techniques, we can disprove Brittle Bone Disease and give patients the resources they need to live their lives to the fullest, despite the challenges the condition presents..

Chapter 2: Holistic Approach to Preventing Brittle Bone Disease

Building Strong Bones Through Nutrition

Calcium and vitamin D are the protagonists of the storey when it comes to building healthy bones. Calcium is the main mineral that gives our bones their strength and structure. In addition to aiding bone growth during childhood, it aids in maintaining bone density into maturity. On the other hand, calcium absorption and utilisation require vitamin D. If we are vitamin D insufficient, our systems cannot properly absorb and utilise the calcium we consume. It's essential to make sure we consume enough of both nutrients as a result.

In order to achieve our calcium demands, it is advisable to incorporate foods high in calcium in our normal diet. Excellent sources of calcium include milk, yoghurt, cheese, and other dairy products. If you are lactose intolerant or follow a plant-based diet, there are numerous calcium-containing foods that are not dairy-based. Leafy green vegetables like kale, collard greens, and broccoli are the finest choices. Additional calcium-rich foods include almonds, tofu, and canned fish with bones like sardines and salmon. By varying our meal options, we may make sure we are consuming an adequate amount of calcium from a range of sources.

Along with calcium, vitamin D is crucial for sustaining the health of bones. Since our bodies can naturally synthesise vitamin D when the sun's UV rays hit our skin, sunlight is the main source of this vitamin. However, factors including our location, skin pigmentation, and limited exposure to sunshine may prevent us from obtaining adequate vitamin D through this method alone. In such cases, it may be vital to look at alternative solutions.

Consuming foods that are fortified with vitamin D or that are naturally high in the vitamin can enhance vitamin D consumption. Among the fatty fish that are an excellent supply of this necessary mineral are salmon, mackerel, and tuna. Eating egg yolks and dairy products with added vitamin D, such as milk and yoghurt, can also help us consume more vitamin D. Speak with a healthcare physician before relying exclusively on dietary sources for vitamin D supplementation.

Even while calcium and vitamin D are in the forefront of the battle for strong bones, we must not minimise the importance of other micronutrients. For instance, magnesium aids in the body's ability to absorb calcium and contributes to the mineralization of bones. Magnesium is abundant in nuts, seeds, legumes, whole grains, and leafy green vegetables.

Phosphorus, another mineral that is abundant in our bones and works in conjunction with calcium to keep our bones strong and healthy. Whole grains, meat, fish, poultry, dairy products, and other animal products are the best sources of phosphorus. A balance must be maintained, though, as an excess of phosphorus might limit calcium absorption.

The health of bones has also been linked to omega-3 fatty acids in addition to these essential minerals. These healthy fats can be found in oily fish like salmon, mackerel, and sardines as well as flaxseeds and chia seeds. They have anti-inflammatory qualities in addition to supporting bone strength and density.

As part of a comprehensive plan for growing strong bones, it's essential to consider both what we consume and how we eat. A healthy relationship with food can be fostered by the practise of mindful eating, which involves being aware of our bodies' signals of hunger and fullness. This style of thinking encourages us to choose nutrient-dense foods that nourish our bodies rather than relying on processed or convenience foods that may be low in essential vitamins and minerals.

It's also crucial to realise that excellent bone health cannot be guaranteed by good eating. Regular exercise, which includes lifting weights, and strength training are also essential. These activities support bone development and bone strength. So let's keep in mind to prioritise providing our bodies with the nutrition they need while also including a well-rounded physical programme into our lives.

In this subsection, we examined the function that nutrition plays in the formation of strong bones. By include calcium-rich foods, ensuring we receive adequate vitamin D, and embracing a mix of micronutrients, we may help our bodies maintain perfect bone health. However, it's important to remember that building strong bones requires a multifaceted approach that includes not only diet but also activity and a holistic approach to wellness. With this knowledge, we may discover the best path to robust, healthy bones and live a fulfilling life.

Exercise and Physical Activity for Bone Strength

In this section, I'll talk about how important physical activity is for strengthening bones and offer tips and suggestions for safe and effective workout routines. But before delving into the specifics, let's first understand the history and idea of brittle bone disease.

Osteogenesis imperfecta (OI), also referred to as brittle bone disease, is a genetic condition marked by fragile bones that are prone to breaking. This condition affects collagen production, a protein required for bone strength and shape. People with OI typically experience fractures as a result, even with minimal bone trauma or stress.

Now, you might be wondering how exercise and physical activity could help a condition that makes bones so brittle. The fundamental premise of Wolff's law, however, holds the solution. In accordance with this principle, external stressors cause bones to strengthen and adapt. In other words, our bones become stronger over time as they adapt to the strain of weight-bearing activities by increasing their mineral content and density.

For those with brittle bone disease, finding the right balance between strengthening their bones and lowering their risk of fractures is critical. Here are some tips and suggestions for safe and effective exercise routines:

1. Consult with a healthcare professional: IBefore starting any exercise programme, it's crucial to consult with your healthcare team, which should include your primary care doctor, physical therapist, and orthopaedic specialist. They can ascertain your unique needs and provide guidance on the most appropriate activities for your condition...

2. Choose low-impact exercises: For those who have brittle bone disease, increased stress on the bones from activities like running or leaping raises their risk of fracture. Instead, concentrate on low-impact exercises that provide the benefits of exercise without the drawbacks. Walking, cycling, swimming, and tai chi are examples of low-impact exercises..

3. Incorporate weight-bearing exercises: Weightlifting exercises are crucial for developing strong bones. These activities encourage the production of bones by requiring you to defy gravity while retaining your body weight. For persons with brittle bone disease, weight-bearing movements including walking, dancing, stair climbing, and low-impact aerobics can be adjusted.

4. Strengthening exercises: Increasing muscle strength, which is essential for supporting and stabilising the bones, is the primary objective of strengthening exercises. Include exercises that target the arms, legs, core, and other significant muscle groups. Several examples include the use of resistance bands and exercises like bodyweight squats, push-ups, and planks.

5. Balance and coordination exercises: Patients with brittle bone disease typically experience balance and coordination issues, which increases their risk of breaking bones and falling. Include exercises that improve stability and balance, such as yoga, Pilates, and tai chi. These exercises not only stop falls but also build up the muscles that support the bones by strengthening the ones that surround them.

6. Focus on proper technique and posture: Proper technique and posture are essential for lowering the risk of injury when exercising. Work with a certified physical therapist or personal trainer to ensure you are exercising safely and correctly. They can give you tips on how to stand or sit correctly, how to breathe, and how to modify certain positions to fit your needs.

7. Gradually increase intensity and duration: It's important to start out cautiously and increase your exercise duration and intensity

gradually. This makes it possible for your bones and muscles to adapt and strengthen, which reduces the risk of overuse problems. Aim to perform two or more days of strength training per week in addition to 75 minutes of intense exercise or 150 minutes of moderate exercise (such as brisk walking) (like swimming).

8. Listen to your body: Pay close attention to how your body feels both during and after exercise. If you have any pain, discomfort, or unusual symptoms, stop exercising and consult your healthcare professional. They can help you decide whether you need to change your exercise routine or undergo more tests.

In addition to these helpful suggestions, a well-balanced diet rich in minerals required for bone health is crucial. Make sure to include adequate calcium, vitamin D, and magnesium in your diet, either from food sources or supplements, as directed by your healthcare professional.

Remember to exercise and engage in physical activity with caution and consideration for your own needs and capabilities. Together with your medical team, you can design an activity programme that improves bone strength while lowering your risk of fracture. Keep moving, stay motivated, and put your bone health first for a stronger, healthier future..

Environmental Factors and Bone Health

Even as a young child, I've always had a deep appreciation for nature. I used to spend a lot of time outside, savouring the cool air and the warmth of the sun on my skin. I had no notion that these regular interactions were creating the framework for strong bones. I am a doctor and a health and wellness coach, so I can speak from experience on the significance of environmental influences in maintaining the best possible bone health.

One of the most crucial environmental factors for healthy bones is sun exposure. Sunlight is not only a source of heat and light, but it also plays a critical role in our bodies' production of vitamin D. Strong, robust bones require a lot of calcium, and vitamin D is essential for calcium absorption. Without adequate vitamin D, our bones become brittle and weak, increasing our risk of disorders like brittle bone disease.

Patients who spend most of their time indoors, whether due to their work or lifestyle choices, are regularly seen at my clinic. This lack of solar exposure could have a substantial negative influence on their bone health. I emphasise how important it is for them to have at least 15 to 30 minutes of direct sunlight on a daily basis. This might be as simple as working in the backyard garden or taking a stroll outside during their lunch break. These modest sun exposures significantly lower the incidence of bone-related diseases.

Although it is frequently overlooked, air quality is a crucial element of the environment that significantly affects bone health. The various toxins, allergens, and pollutants in the air we breathe may have an effect on both our respiratory and skeletal systems. According to studies, prolonged exposure to air pollution can lead to a reduction in bone mineral density, which makes our bones more brittle and brittle.

I advise my patients to be mindful of their surroundings and take the necessary precautions to make sure they are breathing clean air frequently. To help the body detoxify, this may entail using air purifiers at home or at work, avoiding heavily polluted areas, and engaging in practises like deep breathing exercises. We can promote an environment that supports strong, healthy bones by prioritising clean air.

Other environmental factors, such the amount of contaminants in our food and water, can also have an affect on bone health. Pesticides, heavy metals, and other potentially harmful substances may enter our systems through the food and water we consume. The delicate mineral balance in our bones could be disturbed by these contaminants, damaging the bone structure.

I continually emphasise to my patients as a health and wellness coach how crucial it is to follow a balanced, organic diet. Eating foods devoid of harmful pesticides and chemicals may reduce our exposure to these contaminants and enhance our bone health. Additionally, I counsel my patients to drink filtered water and to be aware of the source of their water. It is essential to make sure we are drinking clean, safe water if we want to maintain strong, healthy bones.

Other environmental factors, in addition to diet, air quality, and sun exposure, can have an impact on bone health. For instance, environmental stressors that interfere with our sleep cycles include excessive artificial light or noise pollution. Sleep is essential for our body's ability to repair and regenerate, including maintaining bone health.

I routinely give my patients advice on how to create sleep-friendly bedrooms by cutting back on light and noise pollution. This may involve purchasing blackout curtains or eye shades to create a quiet, dark environment conducive to resting as well as using earplugs or white noise machines to block out noise from outside. By placing a high focus on getting a good night's sleep, we support our body's natural healing processes, which include the preservation of strong, healthy bones.

Although it may seem as though environmental influences and bone health have no connection, they do. By paying attention to the amount of sunlight we receive, the quality of the air we breathe, the food and liquids we consume, and the amount of sleep we get, we may create an environment that supports excellent bone health. Increased outdoor activity, a clean, organic diet, and a sleep-friendly atmosphere are just a few examples of small lifestyle adjustments that can have a significant influence on preventing diseases like brittle bone disease.

In conclusion, environmental factors are crucial for maintaining bone health. Sunlight exposure is necessary for the production of vitamin D, which improves calcium absorption and strong, healthy bones. Clean air and a nutritious, organic diet both reduce exposure to harmful pollutants and slow the loss of bone mineral density. Moreover, promoting the body's organic healing procedures—including the maintenance of bone health—by creating a sleep-friendly environment. By considering and giving attention to these environmental factors, we can take preventative actions to avoid Brittle Bone Disease and assure healthy and robust bones for life...

Lifestyle Modifications for Stronger Bones

A key lifestyle change for stronger bones is giving up smoking. Smoking has long been linked to a higher risk of bone fractures and osteoporosis. Research indicates that smoking negatively affects bone health by reducing bone mineral density and obstructing bone development. Nicotine and other dangerous substances included in cigarettes can directly destroy the cells responsible for creating and maintaining healthy bones. Smoking also reduces the absorption of calcium, a mineral important for healthy bones.

If you want to successfully stop smoking, you must make a detailed plan. It is important to choose a quit date, identify potential smoking triggers, and seek out support from friends and family or even a professional smoking cessation programme. Utilizing nicotine replacement therapy, like as nicotine patches or gum, can also help with the management of withdrawal symptoms. The process of quitting smoking and the desire to smoke can both be aided by finding alternative stress-relieving activities, such as exercising or practising deep breathing.

Another crucial lifestyle adjustment for stronger bones is the restriction of alcohol consumption. Alcohol abuse has been linked to an increased risk of osteoporosis. Alcohol inhibits the body's ability to absorb calcium and vitamin D, both of which are essential for maintaining strong bones. Additionally, it disrupts the hormonal balance required for bone remodelling, which results in a loss of bone mass.

In order to minimise consumption, it is essential to understand how much alcohol is beneficial. Men should generally limit their alcohol consumption to no more than two drinks per day, while women should stick to no more than one. A standard drink is described as having 14 grammes of pure alcohol, thus it's important to be mindful of the drink's size as well. People can reduce their alcohol use by using a variety of strategies, such as goal-setting, tracking their alcohol intake, and making healthier substitutions.

Stress management is a crucial aspect of lifestyle adjustments for stronger bones. Persistent stress has been related to an increased risk of osteoporosis and bone fractures. Stress results in the release of the hormone cortisol, which, in high concentrations, can lead to bone loss. Additionally, stress can lead to unhealthy coping mechanisms like binge drinking or making poor dietary choices, all of which weaken bones.

The detrimental effects of stress on bone health can be considerably reduced by using techniques for controlling stress. These techniques might involve engaging in fun activities, yoga, deep breathing exercises, journaling, or mindfulness meditation. It's critical to identify what works for each person and incorporate these strategies into a regular self-care routine.

Along with the specific lifestyle adjustments outlined above, maintaining a healthy lifestyle generally is essential for stronger bones. It is impossible to stress how important regular exercise is for maintaining bone density and avoiding bone loss. Weight-bearing exercises, such as running, walking, or strength training, have been demonstrated to be very beneficial for bone health. A healthy diet rich in calcium, vitamin D, and other essential nutrients is also necessary for optimum bone strength. Getting enough sleep is essential for the body's natural bone remodelling and repair processes. Last but not least, maintaining strong bones necessitates that you maintain a healthy body weight and avoid severe diets or weight-loss methods.

For control and prevention of brittle bone disease, one's lifestyle must be improved to support healthier bones. Giving up smoking, drinking less alcohol, and using stress management techniques are important components of these changes. It is essential to collaborate with a healthcare professional or a team of experts to develop a tailored approach that takes into account specific needs and objectives. Making these lifestyle adjustments and taking care of one's bone health can significantly improve one's bone strength and overall wellbeing...

Preventive Measures for Brittle Bone Disease

Regular Health Check-Ups:

Regular medical checks are essential for persons who are prone to Brittle Bone Disease. By seeing your doctor frequently, you'll be able to see any early warning signs or symptoms and take the appropriate steps to halt any worsening of your condition. During periodic exams, your doctor may assess your overall health, including the state of your bones, and provide you with wise counsel.

One of the most crucial aspects in the health check-up process is discussing your medical history and family history with your healthcare provider. Identification of your brittle bone disease risk factors requires these information. Therefore, it's imperative to provide accurate information about any past fractures, bone conditions, or relatives who have OI...

Bone Density Screenings:

Examinations of bone density are an essential part in preventing brittle bone disease. These screenings employ the non-invasive dual-energy x-ray absorptiometry (DXA) technique to measure bone density. By evaluating your bone density, medical professionals can identify any anomalies or signs of low bone density suggestive of OI.

Bone density examinations are frequently indicated for people who have a higher risk of developing OI, such as those who have multiple fractures or a family history of the condition. These tests allow medical experts to monitor the progression of the illness and alter treatment plans as appropriate...

Genetic Counseling:

Genetic counselling is a vital component of treatment for brittle bone disease prevention. It requires scheduling a consultation with a licenced genetic counsellor who can assess your risk of OI based on your genes and family history. In addition to discussing OI's inheritance patterns, the counsellor will provide information on the possibility that the condition will be passed on to following generations.

During a genetic counselling session, you can learn more about the specific type of OI that runs in your family and the risks associated with it. In order to ascertain if you have the genes that cause OI or not, the counsellor will also go over the diagnostic techniques that are available, such as genetic testing.

In addition, genetic counselling offers psychological support to individuals and families who are at risk for OI. The counsellor can guide you through the decision-making process if you plan to have children by discussing options like prenatal diagnosis or pre-implantation genetic diagnosis to lower the possibility of passing on the issue.

It's crucial to understand that genetic counselling can benefit everyone, not just people who already have OI. This is true whether or not there is a known family history of the disorder. With the aid of genetic counsellors, a newly developing mutation that might affect future generations can be detected.

Lifestyle Modifications:

In addition to medical treatments, making specific lifestyle modifications can significantly help avoid Brittle Bone Disease. These adjustments also reduce the risk of fractures while enhancing bone health.

A diet rich in calcium and vitamin D that is well-balanced is essential for maintaining strong, healthy bones. Calcium is a crucial mineral that supports the development and maintenance of bone density. The best sources of calcium are dairy products like milk, cheese, and yoghurt, leafy green vegetables, almonds, and fortified foods.

Vitamin D is necessary for the absorption of calcium. The greatest way to get vitamin D is from sunlight, which may be gained by spending time outside. Depending on how much sun exposure you have access to, you might need to take vitamin D supplements or eat foods that have been fortified with it.

Regular exercise is essential for maintaining strong bones. Weight-bearing workouts that stimulate the bones and help to maintain bone density include weightlifting, jogging, dancing, and walking. You should seek the advice of a physical therapist or other healthcare professional to develop an exercise programme that is tailored to your particular needs and abilities.

Additionally important is avoiding situations or actions that increase the risk of fractures or falls. By adopting precautions, such as removing tripping hazards, using assistive devices when necessary, and maintaining enough lighting in your house, the risk of bone injuries can be significantly decreased.

Counseling and Psychological Techniques:

The physical and mental demands of having brittle bone disease can be high. Therefore, preventive interventions should go beyond the realm of the physical and include psychological counselling and methods in order to support those who are at risk for or have been diagnosed with OI.

Using coping methods, people with OI can manage their emotional well-being. Utilizing practises like mindfulness, meditation, and breathing exercises can help people with the disease by reducing the stress and worry that are usually associated to it. Additionally, counselling can provide a safe space for discussing emotions and challenges related to OI, enabling people to travel their paths with a better support network.

Overall, preventing Brittle Bone Disease requires an all-encompassing approach that includes regular physicals, bone density tests, genetic counselling, dietary adjustments, and psychological support. By using these preventive measures, people can significantly reduce their risk of developing OI and enhance their overall quality of life.

I implore everyone, especially those who are at danger, to take these preventive measures seriously. I practise medicine and work as a wellness consultant. Keep in mind that prevention is always better to treatment and that by equipping ourselves with the right knowledge and resources, we may enhance our general health and wellness..

Chapter 3: Managing Brittle Bone Disease

Fracture Prevention and First Aid

People with brittle bone disease frequently fracture because of the weakening and brittleness of their bones. Even very slight trauma or stress can cause fractures, which can be extremely painful, incapacitating, and even lethal. Because of this, it is crucial for those who have this illness to take precautions to prevent fractures and to be knowledgeable about first aid procedures in case a fracture does happen.

This chapter's subchapter contains comprehensive instructions on fracture prevention techniques that can significantly lower the risk of fractures. Understanding that brittle bone disease is a condition for which prevention is always preferable than treatment is essential.

Being healthy is the first and most crucial step towards preventing fractures. A diet that is well-balanced, rich in calcium, vitamin D, and other essential minerals is vital for bone building and preservation. Regular exercise that emphasises building strength, flexibility, and balance is also crucial. However, you should consult a healthcare professional before starting any fitness programme because they may suggest which workouts are safe and appropriate for your situation.

It is important to keep in mind that particular movements and activities can significantly increase the risk of fractures. Patients with brittle bone disease should avoid contact sports, high-impact activities, and any movements that put undue strain on their bones. As a health and wellness coach, I work closely with individuals to assist them in identifying and modifying dangerous behaviours. Making simple changes and looking for other ways to stay active can help us reduce the risk of fractures.

In addition to modifying one's lifestyle, there are a number of environmental policies that can be put in place to prevent fractures. It is essential to offer a friendly and safe living space. This means removing trip hazards, utilising non-slip mats in the bathroom, installing grab bars, and ensuring that there is adequate illumination throughout the entire house. These minor changes significantly reduce the frequency of accidental falls and the resulting fractures.

I can't overstate how crucial regular medical visits are for those with Brittle Bone Disease. Medical professionals can monitor bone density and overall bone health during these checks, identify any potential issues, and take appropriate action before fractures occur. One example of a cutting-edge imaging technique that can provide vital information to guide treatment and preventive measures is a bone density scan.

However, despite all of our efforts, fractures could still occur. As a result, it is equally important for patients with Brittle Bone Disease to be familiar with first aid techniques in order to effectively manage fractures. In this chapter's subsections, I'll go over how to handle a fracture until aid arrives.

The first and most crucial step is to remain calm and reassuring for the fractured person. Panic will only worsen the situation and cause unneeded stress and suffering. By retaining your composure, you can show solidity and calm the person's anxiousness.

The injured limb must next be immobilised to prevent further damage. To support the injured area gently, use your hands or any soft padding, such as towels or cloths. Avoid attempting to realign the bones if they are plainly out of place because doing so could cause further injury. Instead, focus on providing consolation until emergency help arrives.

If there are any open wounds or bleeding, it must be stopped. Gently press the area with a clean towel or sterile bandage to aid in halting the bleeding. Always prioritise your own safety by donning gloves or erecting a barrier between you and the injured person, especially if there's a potential you might come in contact with bodily fluids.

If they are not contraindicated for the person, nonsteroidal anti-inflammatory drugs (NSAIDs) or over-the-counter painkillers may be used for pain management. Before administering any medication, a healthcare professional should be consulted, especially if the patient is already taking another prescription or has underlying medical conditions.

Throughout the entire process, communication is crucial. Maintain constant contact with emergency medical services, provide them with up-to-date information regarding the fracture, and follow their instructions until help arrives. If they have more information, they can better prepare to provide the necessary medical assistance.

In conclusion, effective treatment of brittle bone disease depends on preventing fractures and providing basic medical care. By altering their behaviours, safeguarding their environment, and taking extra precautions, people with this illness can significantly reduce their chance of fractures. Knowledge of first aid techniques is also essential to ensuring prompt and appropriate care in the event of a fracture. By equipping ourselves with the knowledge and skills to prevent and treat fractures, we can help persons with Brittle Bone Disease lead complete lives..

Assistive Devices and Adaptive Equipment

Throughout history, people have been seeking ways to become more independent and mobile. Because of advancements in adapted equipment and assistive technologies, people with varied degrees of physical disability are now leading better lives. The earliest known usage of assistive technology was the use of wooden canes to assist those who had mobility issues in ancient Egypt.

Over the years, technology has advanced swiftly, leading to the development of numerous assistive devices and adaptable equipment. Today, a wide range of instruments are easily accessible and each is tailored to certain needs and purposes. Let's have a look at some of the most common assistive devices that sufferers of brittle bone disease employ.

1. Wheelchairs:

One of the most well-known and widely used assistive technology is the wheelchair. When using wheelchairs, people with Brittle Bone Disease are more independent. They come in a range of designs, including manual wheelchairs that the user propels themselves in using their upper body strength and battery-powered motorised wheelchairs. It is crucial to choose a wheelchair that meets the needs of the user in terms of support, comfort, and lifestyle.

2. Walkers:

Walkers are an essential aid for people with Brittle Bone Disease, particularly for those who still have some degree of mobility. By offering stability and support, walkers lower the danger of falls and fractures when moving about. Among the several varieties of walkers that are offered are rollators, wheeled walkers, and standard walkers. Which type of walker the user should use will depend on their level of mobility and balance.

3. Canes:

Canes are a popular option for those with Brittle Bone Disease who just require a little assistance. They help with stability and weight distribution while walking, which lowers the strain on brittle bones. Straight, quad, and offset canes are just a few of the many diverse cane styles. The kind of cane to employ will depend on the user's balance and stability requirements.

4. Stairlifts:

Stairlifts are a fantastic option for those with Brittle Bone Disease who have problems climbing stairs. People may easily transition between levels thanks to these devices, which are located on staircases. There are straight stairlifts for straight staircases and curved stairlifts for spiral or curved staircases. They can be modified to meet various stairway configurations and user requirements.

5. Ramps:

Ramps provide a safer and more practical alternative for people with brittle bone disease who use mobility aids like wheelchairs or walkers to navigate stairs or elevation changes. Ramps can be installed at home entrances, walkways, or public places to facilitate wheelchair accessible. The ramps must meet accessibility standards and be designed with the user's particular needs in mind.

6. Bed and Bath Safety Equipment:

Accessible bathroom and bedroom equipment and aids can greatly increase independence and safety for those with brittle bone disease. Bed rails, for instance, provide help and security when getting in and out of bed. Bathroom safety equipment like grab bars, shower chairs, and raised toilet seats help people maintain stability and reduce the risk of falling.

7. Orthotics and Prosthetics:

Orthotics and prosthetics are devices that provide support and replace missing or weak body parts. Examples of orthotics include braces and splints, which help to stabilise unstable joints and avoid fractures. Contrarily, prostheses are substitute limbs for missing body parts that keep persons with Brittle Bone Disease mobile and independent. Both orthotics and prosthetics require specialised fitting and customization for each user.

8. Communication and Assistive Technology:

In addition to physical aids, people with Brittle Bone Disease have access to a wide range of communication and assistive technology alternatives. With the use of these devices, people can overcome challenges with communication, speech, hearing, and vision. Software for reading on screens, hearing aids, magnifying glasses, and speech-generating apparatus are a few examples.

Getting and using adaptive equipment and assistive technology can occasionally be scary given the large range of options available. It is imperative to consult a medical professional, such as an occupational therapist or physical therapist, who specialises in treating patients with Brittle Bone Disease. Depending on the person's level of mobility and specific needs, these professionals can assess their requirements and offer suggestions.

In addition to speaking with healthcare professionals, there are several options available for locating assistive technology and equipment that has been modified. Thanks to the range of options provided by online medical supply stores and specialty sellers, people can assess numerous brands and models. Some insurance policies and government programmes may also cover these devices or make you eligible for financial aid.

It's crucial to remember that assistive technology and adapted equipment are instruments that increase independence and mobility. However, they do not restrict or categorise a person's potential or abilities. With the right assistance, people with brittle bone disease can live happy lives and achieve their goals. By utilising assistive technology and adapted equipment, they can overcome physical limitations and celebrate their tenacity and fortitude.

In conclusion, enhancing independence and mobility in patients with brittle bone disease requires the use of assistive technologies and specially designed equipment. Wheelchairs, walkers, communication aids, and ramps are just a few of the many equipment that are available to meet specific needs. It is essential to consult with medical professionals and investigate various resources to find the finest answers. Patients with Brittle Bone Disease can use assistive technologies to manage their everyday lives with confidence, maintain their dignity, and achieve their goals...

Pain Management Strategies

Pharmacological Approaches:

The pain caused by Brittle Bone Disease may be effectively managed with pharmaceutical therapies. These medications function to improve overall comfort while reducing pain and inflammation. Because every patient is unique, the medication chosen should be based on their individual needs and circumstances. Here are a few popular medicinal treatments:

1. Analgesics: Acetaminophen and nonsteroidal anti-inflammatory drugs (NSAIDs), such as ibuprofen, are analgesic medications that can help manage the mild to moderate pain brought on by Brittle Bone Disease. By lowering inflammation and pain, these medications provide patients a break.

2. Opioids: When there is extreme pain, the doctor might advise using opioids. Opioids like oxycodone and morphine have a powerful analgesic effect, but they also come with the danger of dependence and side effects. Working closely with the patient's healthcare team is crucial for monitoring and controlling the patient's opioid use.

3. Antidepressants: Two antidepressant drug families, tricyclic antidepressants and selective serotonin reuptake inhibitors (SSRIs), can also help manage the chronic pain brought on by brittle bone disease. These medications alter the chemistry of the brain to reduce the intensity of pain sensations.

4. Antiepileptic Drugs: Controlling the nerve-related pain brought on by Brittle Bone Disease may benefit from the use of antiepileptic medications like gabapentin and pregabalin, which are widely prescribed to treat seizures. These drugs provide patients with relief by calming down overactive nerve signals.

It is essential to consult a healthcare provider before starting any pharmacological intervention. Based on your medical history, current medications, and any potential side effects, they can advise you on the best course of action..

Non-Pharmacological Approaches:

In addition to pharmaceutical treatments, non-pharmacological techniques can significantly aid persons with Brittle Bone Disease in controlling their pain. These approaches emphasise holistic and complementary therapies that work in tandem with prescription medications to lessen pain and improve overall wellbeing. Here are a few effective natural cures:

1. Physical Therapy: Physical therapy frequently helps to relieve pain associated with brittle bone disease. A skilled physical therapist can design a unique exercise regimen that emphasises balance, strength, and flexibility. These exercises minimise pain by building stronger muscles and bones, which reduces the risk of fractures.

2. Occupational Therapy: Modifying the surroundings and daily routines in order to decrease pain and promote function is the major objective of occupational therapy. An occupational therapist can evaluate the patient's particular needs and recommend assistance, modifications, and adaptable techniques to reduce discomfort and enhance quality of life...

3. Relaxation Techniques: The fact that stress and concern can make pain seem worse highlights the significance of adding relaxation techniques in the pain treatment regimen. A few approaches that can reduce pain and promote relaxation include deep breathing exercises, guided visualisation, meditation, and progressive muscle relaxation.

4. Heat and Cold Therapy: Applying heat or ice to hurting areas might provide momentary comfort and reduce inflammation. Examples of heat treatments that can aid in relaxing muscles and easing discomfort include warm baths or heating pads. Ice packs or cold compresses can be used as a cold treatment to reduce swelling and edoema and numb the affected area..

5. Transcutaneous Electrical Nerve Stimulation (TENS): TENS is a non-invasive technique that uses low-voltage electrical currents to stimulate nerve fibres, sending information to the brain that can help block or reduce pain signals. TENS devices can be used by patients at home with the assistance of a healthcare professional. TENS equipment is portable.

6. Massage Therapy: Massage therapy aids in stress reduction, soothes tense muscles, and lessens brittle bone pain. A certified massage therapist with additional training in treating osteoporosis patients can provide targeted strategies for comfort improvement and pain management.

It is imperative to remember that a person's comprehensive pain management plan should incorporate non-pharmacological techniques in addition to medication and other treatments. Working together with a multidisciplinary healthcare team that consists of physical therapists, occupational therapists, and complementary therapists helps ensure a thorough approach to pain management for Brittle Bone Disease.

Finally, people with Brittle Bone Disease need to appropriately manage their pain. With the help of both pharmaceutical and non-pharmacological techniques, patients can get rid of their pain, lessen inflammation, and improve their overall quality of life. Working together with a healthcare team and exploring various methods will help patients find a customised pain management plan that suits their unique needs and circumstances..

Psychological Support and Coping Strategies

Living with brittle bone disease can be very challenging, both physically and mentally. The limitations of the condition and continued fracture risk might lead to higher levels of anxiety, stress, and even despair. I think that providing holistic healthcare means not just considering the physical aspects of a disease but also the patient's emotional and psychological well-being. As a medical professional and wellness coach, I say this. In this section, I'll provide you some advice and coping techniques to help you cope with the psychological challenges that come with brittle bone disease.

Mental Health Considerations:

The psychosocial impact of brittle bone disease cannot be disregarded. People with this condition usually experience heightened levels of worry and despondency because of the ongoing discomfort, limited mobility, and dread of fractures. Recognizing and addressing these mental health disorders is crucial in order to offer comprehensive care.

Priority should be given to recognising the emotional toll that brittle bone disease takes. It's normal to experience periodic feelings of fatigue, annoyance, or even despair. But it's crucial to keep in mind that you shouldn't let these bad emotions rule you. I encourage patients to express their views honestly and freely, whether it be by writing, speaking to a trustworthy friend or family member, or seeing a therapist. Keep in mind that acknowledging and understanding your feelings is the first step toward healing..

Resilience-Building Techniques:

The key to managing any chronic condition is building resilience. It requires developing the mental toughness required to go through the challenges Brittle Bone Disease presents. Here are some techniques for increasing resilience that might be effective:

1. Mindfulness and Meditation: By practising mindfulness and meditation, people with brittle bone disease can learn to cultivate a sense of tranquilly and inner peace. These techniques help people to focus on the present moment rather than worrying about what the future may hold. This has the potential to be very helpful for managing anxiety and reducing stress..

2. Positive Self-Talk: Our internal dialogue has a big impact on our mental health. People with brittle bone disease can become happier by being encouraged to use positive self-talk. Affirmations like "I am strong," "I am capable," and "I am resilient" can be repeated to remind oneself of one's inner strength and ability to overcome obstacles.

3. Developing a Supportive Mindset: It is essential to be in a supportive and upbeat environment. Having a support system of family, friends, and medical professionals who understand your challenges and provide encouragement can have a big impact on your psychological welfare. Remember that you are not alone in your journey.

4. Seeking Professional Help: It's possible that increasing resilience won't always be enough. Receiving professional treatment through counselling or therapy can be quite beneficial in these circumstances. A mental health expert may assist patients with Brittle Bone Disease in navigating their emotions and successfully managing their mental health with the support of coping methods and other techniques.

The Importance of Social Support Networks:

One of the most crucial aspects of controlling brittle bone disease is having a strong social support network. Family, friends, and medical professionals can all be of considerable emotional and practical support to those with this disease.

It can be highly beneficial to participate in support groups created especially for those with brittle bone disease. In these groups, people can open up about their experiences, concerns, and coping techniques in a supportive setting with others who can genuinely connect to them. Developing relationships with others who are aware of the unique challenges of living with brittle bone disease can make patients feel less alone and more a part of the community.

Additionally, it's crucial to be open and truthful with loved ones about your preferences and limitations. If they are aware of Brittle Bone Disease, they can better understand its implications and provide the appropriate support. Family and friends may be very beneficial in creating a climate that is encouraging and supportive of emotional well-being..

Conclusion:

As crucial as addressing the physical symptoms of Brittle Bone Disease is managing its psychological effects. Individuals with this illness can set out on a journey of emotional recovery and well-being by acknowledging mental health considerations, putting resilience-building skills into practise, and embracing social support networks. Remember that you are more than your diagnosis, and that you can face the difficulties of brittle bone disease with courage and optimism if you have the necessary resources and support.

We will go into more detail about the value of lifestyle changes in managing brittle bone disease in the following chapter, including nutrition, exercise, and self-care. These factors have a crucial role in enhancing the general health and wellbeing of people with this illness. Stay tuned for insightful analysis and helpful advice to improve your quality of life.

Enhancing Quality of Life

Adaptive leisure is a crucial component of raising the quality of life for people with brittle bone disease. I can speak from experience when I say that engaging in adaptive recreational activities can benefit my patients as a doctor and health and wellness coach. Adaptive recreation is the practise of altering leisure pursuits so that people with impairments can participate in and enjoy them.

Physical activity might be difficult for those with Brittle Bone Disease because of the possibility of fractures. However, people can participate in safe yet pleasurable activities with the right assistance and instruction. Adaptive sports, such power soccer, seated volleyball, and wheelchair basketball, let people develop their strength and coordination while also enjoying the excitement of competition. Yoga and adaptive swimming are two more activities that can enhance flexibility and balance while lowering the incidence of fractures.

Working with a team of specialists from many health and wellness disciplines is crucial to ensuring the security and efficacy of adaptive leisure activities. Physical therapists and occupational therapists that have a focus on adaptive sports and leisure activities collaborate in an interdisciplinary approach. These experts may offer individualised advice, create customised training regimens, and make sure people are utilising adaptive equipment that is appropriate for their particular needs. Together, we can provide a welcoming environment that encourages exercise, social engagement, and personal development.

Vocational rehabilitation is a crucial component of improving the quality of life for people with brittle bone disease. This entails offering people the knowledge and assistance they need to find fulfilling work. People who have brittle bone disease may have particular problems at work, but with the correct support and accommodations, they can succeed in their professions.

The first step in vocational rehabilitation is a thorough evaluation of a person's skills, passions, and objectives. This evaluation assists in determining appropriate career options and potential workplace adjustments that can be made to meet the demands of the individual. Modifications to the workplace could include adjustable timetables, assistive technology, and ergonomic furnishings. In some circumstances, people may also gain advantage from work coaching and training programmes that give them the skills they need to succeed in their chosen profession.

Self-care routines are essential for improving the general quality of life for people with brittle bone disease, in addition to adaptive recreation and vocational rehabilitation. Self-care is defined as practising behaviours that advance one's physical, mental, and emotional wellbeing. It entails setting aside time for oneself, controlling stress, eating a balanced diet, and engaging in mindfulness and relaxation exercises.

Regular stretching exercises to preserve flexibility, check-ups with medical specialists to monitor bone density and general health, and the use of assistive devices and equipment to prevent injuries are all examples of self-care activities for people with Brittle Bone Disease. A higher quality of life can also result from doing things that make you happy and fulfilled, such developing a hobby, spending time with loved ones, and learning self-compassion.

For people with brittle bone disease, coping mechanisms are a crucial component of self-care. Having a chronic illness can be emotionally taxing, so it's critical to learn effective coping skills. These can include developing a positive outlook, going to therapy or counselling, and asking friends, family, or support groups for assistance. People can improve their general health and quality of life by understanding and addressing the emotional components of having brittle bone disease.

In summary, improving the quality of life for people with brittle bone disease requires a holistic strategy that includes self-care routines, adaptive recreation, and vocational rehabilitation. We can enable people to lead satisfying and meaningful lives by giving them the chance to participate in recreational activities, supporting their employment objectives, and encouraging self-care habits. It is my passion to accompany people with Brittle Bone Disease on their road to enhanced quality of life as a physician and health and wellness coach..

Chapter 4: Complementary and Alternative Therapies

Acupuncture and Traditional Chinese Medicine

Traditional Chinese medicine (TCM) has been used as a holistic method of treating a variety of diseases and reestablishing the body's natural balance for thousands of years. One of the main practises in TCM, acupuncture, involves inserting tiny needles into the body at certain sites to promote Qi, or energy flow. An imbalance or obstruction in the flow of Qi, according to this traditional practise, might result in health issues.

According to research, acupuncture may improve bone health and lower the incidence of fractures in people with brittle bone disease. Studies have shown that acupuncture enhances the production of some naturally occurring chemicals, such as serotonin and endorphins, which are essential for bone metabolism. These chemicals support bone repair, decrease pain, and boost bone density.

Researchers from the China Academy of Chinese Medical Sciences looked into how acupuncture affected postmenopausal women with osteoporosis, a disorder closely related to Brittle Bone Disease, and their bone mineral density (BMD). The findings showed that frequent acupuncture sessions significantly increased BMD, suggesting that acupuncture has promise as a non-pharmacological strategy for enhancing bone health.

Acupuncture has also been shown to have a body-wide anti-inflammatory impact. Chronic inflammation can have a negative impact on bone health, causing bone tissues to deteriorate and increasing the risk of fractures. Acupuncture helps maintain and strengthen bones, increasing their resilience, by lowering inflammation.

According to TCM, the body's Yin and Yang energies are out of balance, which leads to brittle bone disease. Yang stands for the energetic and hot qualities, while Yin stands for the nourishing and chilling aspects. Yin and Yang must be in harmony in order to preserve general health, including bone health, according to TCM principles. The goal of acupuncture is to reestablish this balance and advance the person's general wellbeing.

TCM uses herbal treatment in addition to acupuncture to enhance bone health. Over the years, numerous herbal formulas have been created to address various health issues, including problems with the bones. These herbal medicines are well-known for their capacity to strengthen the entire skeletal system and nourish the bones while also enhancing bone density.

Eucommia bark is a common herb for bone health in TCM. Natural substances that have been demonstrated to promote bone growth and prevent bone resorption are abundant in eucommia. It has historically been used to cure ailments like osteoporosis and fractures. Another herb, Chinese angelica root, is well known for its capacity to enhance bone health by nourishing blood and encouraging bone marrow development.

In TCM, nutrition and food are equally important in preventing and treating brittle bone disease. TCM principles state that some foods contain qualities that can improve bone health. For instance, calcium-rich foods like tofu, sesame seeds, and leafy greens are thought to support bone density and nourish the bones. The Yang energy, which is essential for maintaining bone health, is also believed to be strengthened by foods with warming qualities like ginger and cinnamon.

TCM also stresses the significance of modifying one's lifestyle to support bone health. Patients with Brittle Bone Disease are frequently advised to practise Tai Chi and Qi Gong in addition to acupuncture and herbal treatment. These simple workouts lower the risk of falls and fractures by enhancing balance, coordination, and flexibility.

For those with Brittle Bone Disease, incorporating acupuncture and TCM into the therapy regimen can provide a comprehensive and all-encompassing approach to bone health. These activities have the potential to increase bone density, lower the risk of fractures, and enhance quality of life by addressing the underlying bodily imbalances and promoting general wellbeing.

Acupuncture and TCM should not be used in isolation to treat brittle bone disease, it is crucial to remember this. They ought to be incorporated within a whole therapy strategy that also includes prescription drugs, physical activity, and dietary adjustments. To ensure a secure and efficient approach to treating the disease, it is essential to speak with a certified TCM practitioner and collaborate with your medical team.

In conclusion, those with Brittle Bone Disease may benefit from acupuncture and traditional Chinese medicine. These age-old techniques work to correct the body's underlying imbalances while promoting bone repair and energy flow. Acupuncture and Traditional Chinese Medicine (TCM) can help improve bone health, decrease fractures, and increase general well-being when used in conjunction with appropriate medical treatment and lifestyle changes..

Herbal Remedies and Supplements

Introduction:

I firmly believe in the ability of natural cures and supplements to improve our general wellbeing and advance bone health because I practise holistic healthcare. This section will examine a variety of herbal treatments and dietary supplements with potential benefits for bone health. We will examine the available scientific information, safety issues, and possible interactions with common prescription drugs.

1. Ginkgo Biloba:

Popular herbal supplement ginkgo biloba has been used for many years in traditional medicine. It is renowned for its blood flow-improving and antioxidant qualities. Recent research suggests that ginkgo biloba may improve bone health by boosting bone mineral density and decreasing bone loss. It has also been demonstrated to have anti-inflammatory properties, which can help in the treatment of illnesses like osteoporosis.

Ginkgo biloba does have some potential side effects, including gastrointestinal discomfort and headaches, and it can interact with some drugs, including blood thinners. Therefore, it is essential to seek advice from a healthcare provider before adding ginkgo biloba to your regimen.

2. Turmeric:

Curcumin, a substance found in the brilliant yellow spice turmeric, which is frequently used in Indian food, has powerful anti-inflammatory and antioxidant qualities. According to studies, curcumin may protect against bone deterioration by preventing the activity of cells that break down bone and encouraging the growth of new bone cells.

Turmeric has been demonstrated to have a wide range of health advantages, including lowering inflammation, enhancing digestion, and maintaining a healthy immune system, in addition to its potential advantages for bone health. Curcumin is, however, poorly absorbed by the body; nonetheless, taking it with black pepper or fat can improve its absorption..

3. Green Tea:

Green tea is a widely consumed beverage that is rich in polyphenols, which are potent antioxidants. Research suggests that green tea may have a protective effect on bone health by stimulating the activity of bone-forming cells and reducing bone loss. Additionally, it has been shown to have anti-inflammatory properties, which can help alleviate symptoms of conditions such as osteoporosis.

Regular consumption of green tea has also been associated with other health benefits, including weight loss, improved heart health, and a reduced risk of certain cancers. However, it is important to note that excessive consumption of green tea may have adverse effects, such as increased heart rate and insomnia, due to its caffeine content.

4. Red Clover:

Red clover is a flowering plant that has been used in traditional medicine for its potential estrogen-like effects. It contains compounds called isoflavones, which are known for their bone-protective properties. Studies have shown that red clover may help improve bone mineral density and reduce bone loss, particularly in postmenopausal women.

However, it is important to note that red clover may interact with certain medications, and its use should be avoided by individuals with hormone-sensitive conditions, such as breast cancer. As always, it is crucial to consult with a healthcare professional before incorporating red clover into your routine.

5. Omega-3 Fatty Acids:

Omega-3 fatty acids are essential fats that play a crucial role in supporting overall health. They have been found to have anti-inflammatory properties and can help reduce the risk of chronic diseases, including osteoporosis. Studies have shown that omega-3 fatty acids may help increase bone mineral density and reduce bone loss, particularly in older adults.

Fish oil supplements are a common source of omega-3 fatty acids. However, it is important to choose high-quality supplements that have been tested for purity and are free from contaminants such as heavy metals. Additionally, individuals who are taking blood thinners should consult with a healthcare professional before starting omega-3 fatty acid supplementation.

Conclusion:

Herbal remedies and supplements can be valuable allies in maintaining bone health and overall well-being. However, it is essential to approach them with caution and consult with a healthcare professional before incorporating them into your routine, especially if you are taking any medications or have underlying health conditions. By combining these natural remedies with a balanced diet, regular exercise, and a healthy lifestyle, you can take proactive steps toward supporting your bone health and promoting optimal well-being.

Mind-Body Practices for Pain Management

Before we dive into the details of these practices, let us first understand the underlying mechanisms that make them so powerful in pain management. You see, the connection between the mind and the body is an intricate one, with each influencing the other in a multitude of ways. When we experience pain, it not only affects us physically but also has a significant impact on our mental and emotional well-being. This, in turn, can exacerbate the perception of pain and create a vicious cycle that becomes hard to break.

However, by harnessing the power of the mind through mind-body practices, we can disrupt this cycle and find relief from the often debilitating pain caused by Brittle Bone Disease. Through these practices, we can shift our focus away from the pain itself and instead, cultivate a sense of calm, relaxation, and inner peace. By doing so, we can reduce the intensity of the pain and improve our quality of life.

Let us begin with meditation, a practice that has been used for centuries to quiet the mind and promote a deep sense of inner tranquility. When it comes to pain management, meditation can be a game-changer. By bringing our attention to the present moment and focusing on our breath, we can develop a heightened awareness that allows us to detach ourselves from the pain. This doesn't mean that the pain magically disappears, but rather that it loses its hold over us. Through regular meditation practice, we learn to observe the pain without judgment or resistance, and in doing so, we can diminish its impact on us.

But meditation is not the only mind-body practice that can aid in pain management for Brittle Bone Disease. Yoga, a holistic discipline that combines physical postures, breath control, and meditation, also offers immense benefits in this regard. The gentle movements and stretches involved in yoga are not only effective in improving flexibility and strength but also in reducing pain levels. Certain yoga poses can target specific areas affected by Brittle Bone Disease, helping to alleviate discomfort and promote healing. Additionally, the conscious breathing techniques employed in yoga can enhance relaxation, decrease stress, and provide a sense of relief from the constant pain that many individuals with this condition endure.

Another mind-body practice that has shown significant promise in pain management is guided imagery. This technique involves using one's imagination to create vivid, sensory-rich mental images that evoke feelings of calmness, joy, and well-being. By visualizing soothing scenes and engaging all the senses, we can direct our attention away from the pain and instead focus on positive sensations. Guided imagery can be particularly effective when combined with deep relaxation techniques, as it allows us to enter a state of deep relaxation where the pain becomes less prominent.

Now that we have explored the underlying mechanisms and understood the potential of these mind-body practices, let us move on to the practical techniques for their implementation. Meditation, yoga, and guided imagery are all highly individual practices, and what works best for one person may not necessarily work for another. Therefore, it is crucial to approach these practices with an open mind and experiment to find the techniques that resonate most with us.

When it comes to meditation, one can start by finding a comfortable, quiet space where they can sit or lie down without distraction. Closing the eyes, focusing on the breath, and allowing thoughts to come and go without judgment is a simple yet powerful way to begin. Guided meditations, available in the form of audio recordings or apps, can provide additional support and guidance for beginners. As one gains experience and familiarity with the practice, they can explore different meditation techniques such as mindfulness, loving-kindness, or body scan meditations, all of which can be adapted to specifically address pain.

When it comes to yoga, it is essential to start with gentle and beginner-friendly poses that are suitable for one's physical condition. Consulting with a qualified yoga instructor or healthcare professional familiar with Brittle Bone Disease can ensure that the chosen poses are safe and appropriate. Incorporating breath work, such as deep belly breathing or alternate nostril breathing, during the practice can further enhance relaxation and pain relief. As with meditation, finding what feels good and honoring one's limitations is crucial in experiencing the benefits of yoga.

As for guided imagery, there are numerous resources available in the form of audio recordings or books that provide step-by-step instructions for creating healing imagery. These resources often offer a range of guided imagery scripts tailored to different conditions and ailments, including chronic pain. However, one can also develop their own personalized imagery by visualizing a place or scenario that brings them comfort and peace. Engaging all the senses in the visualization, such as imagining the warmth of the sun on the skin or the scent of a blooming flower, can make the experience even more powerful.

In conclusion, mind-body practices such as meditation, yoga, and guided imagery hold tremendous potential when it comes to managing pain for individuals with Brittle Bone Disease. By harnessing the power of the mind, we can transform our relationship with pain, cultivate a sense of inner peace, and improve our overall well-being. It is my sincerest hope that you find solace and relief through the implementation of these practices, and that they become valuable tools on your journey towards holistic health and wellness. Remember, dear readers, that you have the power within you to transcend pain and embrace a life filled with joy, despite the challenges that may come your way.

Energy Healing Modalities

Energy healing modalities, such as Reiki and therapeutic touch, are based on the principle that the human body has an innate energy that can be harnessed and balanced to promote relaxation, reduce stress, and enhance overall well-being. These techniques involve the practitioner using their hands, either by lightly touching or hovering above the body, to transmit healing energy into the patient's energy field.

Let us first explore Reiki, a Japanese technique commonly used to promote relaxation and stress reduction. Reiki is based on the belief that life force energy flows through every living being. If this energy becomes blocked or imbalanced, it can lead to physical, mental, and emotional distress. By channeling the practitioner's energy through their hands into the patient's body, Reiki aims to restore balance and harmony in the energy field, facilitating the body's natural healing process.

Numerous studies have shown the potential benefits of Reiki for individuals with various health conditions, including chronic pain, anxiety, and depression. For individuals with Brittle Bone Disease, Reiki can offer a complementary approach to managing the physical and emotional stress that often accompanies the condition. By promoting relaxation and reducing stress levels, Reiki can potentially alleviate muscle tension, improve sleep quality, and enhance overall well-being.

However, it is important to note that energy healing modalities like Reiki are not meant to replace traditional medical treatments. Rather, they should be used as a complementary approach to support the individual's holistic well-being. It is crucial for individuals with Brittle Bone Disease to consult with their healthcare team and ensure that Reiki is safely integrated into their overall treatment plan.

Therapeutic touch, another energy healing modality, is similar to Reiki in that it involves the practitioner using their hands to promote healing and relaxation. However, therapeutic touch differs in its approach and technique. It is rooted in the belief that the human body is an energy field that can be influenced by the practitioner's touch and intent. By gently moving their hands above the patient's body, the practitioner can manipulate and balance the patient's energy field, promoting healing and overall well-being.

Research on therapeutic touch has shown promising results in reducing pain, anxiety, and stress in individuals with various health conditions. For individuals with Brittle Bone Disease, therapeutic touch can be particularly beneficial in managing pain and promoting relaxation. By addressing the energy imbalances that may contribute to pain and discomfort, therapeutic touch has the potential to provide a natural, non-invasive method of pain management.

It is important to acknowledge that the effectiveness of energy healing modalities, including Reiki and therapeutic touch, is not solely based on scientific evidence. These modalities are rooted in ancient practices and holistic healing traditions that have been passed down through generations. They work on a subtle level, impacting the energy body and the individual's overall well-being. While scientific research can provide insights and support for the potential benefits of these modalities, there is still much to be understood about the mechanisms by which they work.

In considering the use of energy healing modalities, it is essential to approach them with an open mind and a willingness to explore their potential benefits. However, it is equally important to exercise discernment and seek guidance from qualified practitioners who are experienced in working with individuals with Brittle Bone Disease. The integration of energy healing into one's treatment plan should always be done in collaboration with a healthcare team to ensure safety and efficacy.

In conclusion, energy healing modalities, such as Reiki and therapeutic touch, can offer additional support and promote relaxation, stress reduction, and overall well-being for individuals with Brittle Bone Disease. These techniques, when used in conjunction with traditional medical interventions, have the potential to enhance the quality of life for individuals with chronic conditions. While more research is needed to fully understand the mechanisms and effectiveness of these modalities, the growing body of evidence and the countless testimonials from individuals who have benefited from them cannot be ignored. As we continue to demystify Brittle Bone Disease, it is crucial to embrace a holistic approach that encompasses both conventional medicine and integrative practices. By doing so, we can provide comprehensive care that addresses the physical, emotional, and energetic needs of individuals with Brittle Bone Disease, ultimately supporting their journey to wellness and a fulfilling life.

Integrating Complementary Therapies

When it comes to Brittle Bone Disease, it is important to understand that there is no cure. However, there are several ways to manage the symptoms and improve the quality of life for individuals with this condition. Traditional medical treatments such as medications, physical therapy, and surgery are widely used and play a crucial role in the management of Brittle Bone Disease. However, integrating complementary therapies can provide additional benefits and support to patients.

One of the key aspects of integrating complementary therapies is collaborating with a team of healthcare professionals from different fields. This team may include medical doctors, physical therapists, nutritionists, psychologists, and alternative medicine practitioners. By working together, we can create a customized treatment plan that combines the best of traditional medical treatments with complementary therapies.

Before integrating any complementary therapy, it is important to conduct thorough research and gather evidence-based information. This will help us make informed decisions and choose therapies that have shown promising results in managing the symptoms of Brittle Bone Disease. Gathering research and evidence can be a daunting task, but it is essential to ensure that the therapies we recommend are safe and effective.

Once we have gathered the necessary research and evidence, the next step is to select suitable complementary therapies for each individual. It is important to remember that what works for one person may not work for another. Each individual is unique and may respond differently to various therapies. This is where the expertise of a healthcare professional comes in handy. By carefully assessing the individual's condition, lifestyle, and preferences, we can recommend the most suitable complementary therapies.

Some of the complementary therapies that have shown promise in managing the symptoms of Brittle Bone Disease include acupuncture, herbal medicine, massage therapy, and chiropractic care. These therapies can help alleviate pain, reduce inflammation, promote bone health, and improve overall well-being. However, it is important to note that these therapies should be used alongside traditional medical treatments and not as a substitute for them.

Collaboration with healthcare professionals is crucial throughout the integration process. It is important to keep the lines of communication open and share information with the entire healthcare team. This ensures that everyone is on the same page and that the treatment plan is cohesive and comprehensive. Regular meetings and updates with the healthcare team will help us monitor the progress of the individual and make any necessary adjustments to the treatment plan.

In addition to collaborating with healthcare professionals, it is also essential to involve the individual with Brittle Bone Disease in the decision-making process. They should be educated about the different complementary therapies available and encouraged to voice their preferences and concerns. By actively involving the individual, we can create a sense of empowerment and ensure that they feel heard and supported throughout the treatment journey.

Another important aspect of integrating complementary therapies is educating patients and their families about the potential risks and benefits of these therapies. It is important to provide accurate and evidence-based information, as well as to address any misconceptions or concerns they may have. By providing education and support, we can empower individuals to make well-informed decisions about their treatment plan and actively participate in their own care.

Lastly, it is important to regularly evaluate the integration of complementary therapies and make any necessary adjustments. This can be done through ongoing monitoring of the individual's progress, gathering feedback from the healthcare team, and keeping up with the latest research in the field. By continuously evaluating and adapting the treatment plan, we can ensure that the individual is receiving the most effective and appropriate care.

In conclusion, integrating complementary therapies into the overall treatment plan for Brittle Bone Disease can provide additional benefits and support to patients. By collaborating with healthcare professionals, conducting thorough research, and making informed decisions, we can create a comprehensive and effective treatment plan that combines traditional medical treatments with complementary therapies. By actively involving the individual and their family in the decision-making process, providing education and support, and regularly evaluating and adapting the treatment plan, we can work towards improving the quality of life for individuals with Brittle Bone Disease.

Chapter 5: Nurturing Emotional Well-being

Embracing Self-Acceptance and Body Positivity

Living with Brittle Bone Disease can present unique obstacles and physical limitations, which can often lead to feelings of insecurity, self-doubt, and even self-loathing. However, it is essential to recognize that our bodies are not mere vessels, but rather unique and remarkable entities that deserve love, respect, and acceptance. Embracing self-acceptance and body positivity is a transformative journey that requires a shift in mindset and a commitment to self-care.

The first step in embracing self-acceptance and body positivity is to challenge societal norms and expectations of beauty and perfection. It is important to remember that beauty comes in all shapes, sizes, and abilities. Our worth is not determined by our physical appearance or abilities but by our character, kindness, and resilience. By acknowledging and challenging these societal pressures, we can begin to redefine our own standards of beauty and focus on the qualities that make us unique and exceptional.

One effective way to cultivate self-acceptance and body positivity is through positive self-talk and affirmations. Our thoughts have a powerful impact on our emotions and actions. Therefore, it is crucial to replace negative self-talk with positive affirmations. Encourage yourself, remind yourself of your strengths and accomplishments, and affirm your value as a person beyond your physical limitations. By consistently practicing positive self-talk, you can gradually rewire your mindset and foster self-love and acceptance.

Another essential aspect of embodying self-acceptance and body positivity is embracing self-care practices that prioritize your physical and emotional well-being. Regular exercise, tailored to your specific needs and abilities, can improve muscle strength, flexibility, and overall well-being. Engaging in activities that align with your interests and passions can also boost your self-esteem and sense of purpose. Remember, self-care goes beyond physical health and encompasses emotional and mental well-being as well. Engage in activities that bring you joy, practice mindfulness and relaxation techniques, and seek support from loved ones or a professional therapist when needed.

Additionally, surrounding yourself with a supportive and inclusive community plays a pivotal role in fostering self-acceptance and body positivity. Connect with individuals who understand and appreciate the challenges you face, and who uplift and inspire you. Social media platforms can also be valuable spaces to find support, as there are communities dedicated to promoting body positivity and acceptance. Engage with these communities, share your experiences, and learn from others who have embarked on a similar journey.

Taking care of your mental health is an integral part of embracing self-acceptance and body positivity. Living with Brittle Bone Disease can be emotionally challenging, and it is common to experience feelings of frustration, helplessness, or even sadness. It is vital to acknowledge these emotions and seek professional help when necessary. Therapy, counseling, or support groups can provide a safe space to process your feelings, develop coping strategies, and gain a deeper understanding of yourself and your journey.

Celebrating your accomplishments, no matter how small they may seem, is an essential practice in cultivating self-acceptance and body positivity. Recognize and acknowledge the daily triumphs and milestones you achieve despite the challenges you face. Whether it is overcoming a physical barrier, pursuing your passions, or nurturing meaningful relationships, take pride in your achievements. Each step forward is a testament to your strength and resilience.

Lastly, it is crucial to remember that self-acceptance and body positivity are ongoing journeys. There will be days when self-doubt creeps in, or when you struggle to see your worth beyond your physical limitations. During these moments, be gentle with yourself, practice self-compassion, and remind yourself of the progress you have made. Embrace the ups and downs as a part of your growth and continue to nurture a positive mindset and a deep sense of self-love.

In conclusion, embracing self-acceptance and body positivity is a vital aspect of living a fulfilling life with Brittle Bone Disease. By challenging societal norms, practicing positive self-talk and affirmations, prioritizing self-care, seeking support from a supportive community, taking care of your mental health, celebrating your accomplishments, and embracing the journey of self-acceptance, you can truly thrive and find joy and fulfillment in your unique and exquisite self. Remember, you are beautiful, resilient, and deserving of love and acceptance exactly as you are.

Overcoming Emotional Challenges

Anxiety is a common emotional challenge experienced by individuals with Brittle Bone Disease. The constant fear of fractures and injuries can cause heightened anxiety levels, which may hinder their ability to live a normal life. It is essential to address anxiety head-on and provide individuals with the tools they need to manage it effectively.

One strategy that has proven to be effective in managing anxiety is practicing relaxation techniques. Deep breathing exercises, guided imagery, and progressive muscle relaxation are all techniques that can help individuals with Brittle Bone Disease calm their minds and reduce anxiety levels. By incorporating these techniques into their daily routine, they can develop a sense of control over their anxiety and improve their overall well-being.

Another important aspect of overcoming anxiety is building a support network. Connecting with others who have a similar condition can provide a sense of understanding and shared experiences. Joining support groups or online communities can be beneficial in providing emotional support and encouragement. Additionally, it is essential for individuals with Brittle Bone Disease to have a strong support system of family and friends who can offer emotional support during challenging times.

Depression is another emotional challenge that individuals with Brittle Bone Disease may face. The constant pain, limitations, and challenges associated with the condition can take a toll on one's mental health, leading to feelings of sadness, hopelessness, and low self-esteem. It is crucial to address depression promptly and seek appropriate treatment.

Cognitive-behavioral therapy (CBT) has proven to be effective in managing depression in individuals with chronic conditions. CBT helps individuals challenge negative thought patterns and develop healthier coping strategies. Working with a therapist who specializes in chronic illnesses can provide individuals with the necessary tools to manage their depression effectively.

Self-esteem issues are also common among individuals with Brittle Bone Disease. Constant fractures and physical limitations can make individuals feel insecure about their appearance and abilities. It is essential to address these self-esteem issues and help individuals develop a positive self-image.

One approach to improving self-esteem is through a holistic wellness plan that focuses on overall well-being. By incorporating exercise routines tailored to their abilities, individuals with Brittle Bone Disease can improve their physical strength and overall fitness, which can have a positive impact on their self-confidence. It is important to consult with healthcare professionals and physical therapists to design an exercise plan that is safe and effective.

Additionally, practicing self-compassion and self-acceptance is crucial for individuals with Brittle Bone Disease. Instead of focusing on physical limitations, they can shift their mindset to focus on their strengths and accomplishments. Engaging in activities that bring them joy and fulfillment can also boost self-esteem and overall well-being.

In conclusion, this subchapter has delved into the emotional challenges faced by individuals with Brittle Bone Disease and provided practical strategies for overcoming them. From addressing anxiety through relaxation techniques and building a support network to managing depression with cognitive-behavioral therapy and improving self-esteem through holistic wellness, there are various tools and techniques available to individuals with Brittle Bone Disease to help them overcome these emotional challenges. By implementing these strategies and seeking appropriate support, individuals with Brittle Bone Disease can lead fulfilling lives and achieve emotional well-being despite the challenges they face.

Building Resilience and Mental Strength

In life, we all encounter challenges and setbacks that can test our emotional strength and resilience. Whether it's a major life-changing event or a series of smaller obstacles, these moments can leave us feeling vulnerable and overwhelmed. However, with the right mindset and tools, it is possible to build resilience and mental strength that will enable you to navigate these tough times with grace and confidence.

Here, in this chapter, we will delve deep into the techniques and strategies that can help you build resilience and develop a strong mental foundation. By focusing on mindset shifts, positive affirmations, and mindfulness practices, you will be able to enhance your emotional well-being and develop the inner strength needed to face any adversity that comes your way.

Mindset Shifts: Harnessing the Power of Your Thoughts

Our thoughts have a powerful influence on our emotions, actions, and overall well-being. By understanding and harnessing the power of our thoughts, we can create positive mindset shifts that propel us forward, even in the face of adversity.

One of the key mindset shifts to cultivate resilience is reframing challenges as opportunities for growth. Instead of allowing setbacks to define us, we can reframe them as valuable learning experiences that allow us to become stronger and more resilient individuals. This shift in perspective enables us to reframe negative situations as positive opportunities, helping us to stay motivated and focused on personal growth.

Another important mindset shift is practicing self-compassion. Often, when faced with challenges, we tend to be overly critical of ourselves, which can further exacerbate feelings of stress and helplessness. By adopting a kind and understanding internal dialogue, we can cultivate self-compassion, which in turn allows us to bounce back from difficulties more easily. Instead of berating ourselves for mistakes, we learn to treat ourselves with kindness and understanding, ultimately building our resilience and mental strength.

Positive Affirmations: Empowering Yourself Through Self-Talk

Positive affirmations are an incredibly powerful tool for building resilience and mental strength. By consciously choosing positive and empowering statements to reinforce within ourselves, we can rewire our thought patterns and shift our mindset towards a more positive and resilient outlook.

Within the realm of brittle bone disease, it is important to remind ourselves that our condition does not define us or limit us from pursuing our dreams and aspirations. By repeating affirmations such as "I am resilient and capable of overcoming any obstacle," or "I am fully capable of leading a fulfilling and empowered life despite my condition", we are actively counteracting any negative self-talk that may arise and replacing it with empowering beliefs.

Incorporating these positive affirmations into daily practices, such as reciting them in the morning or before bed, can significantly enhance our ability to navigate the challenges of brittle bone disease with resilience and mental strength. Through consistent repetition, these affirmations become ingrained in our subconscious mind, reinforcing positive thoughts and belief systems.

Mindfulness Practices: Cultivating Emotional Well-Being

Mindfulness practices, such as meditation and deep breathing exercises, are invaluable tools for building resilience and mental strength. By bringing our awareness to the present moment and cultivating a non-judgmental attitude, we can develop emotional well-being and the ability to handle adversity with grace and composure.

One particularly effective mindfulness practice for individuals with brittle bone disease is body scan meditation. This practice involves directing our attention to different parts of the body, observing physical sensations without judgment. By cultivating this non-judgmental awareness, we can develop a deeper connection with our bodies, nurturing a sense of acceptance and compassion for ourselves.

Another mindfulness practice that can enhance resilience is conscious breathing. Taking a few moments each day to focus on our breath, inhaling deeply and exhaling slowly, allows us to activate the body's relaxation response, reducing stress and anxiety. This practice not only calms the mind but also brings us back to the present moment, grounding us in the here and now.

Incorporating mindfulness practices into our daily routine can significantly enhance our ability to cope with the challenges of brittle bone disease. By developing a strong sense of presence and emotional well-being, we become more resilient and better equipped to navigate the ups and downs of life.

Conclusion

Building resilience and mental strength is an ongoing journey that requires consistent effort and practice. By embracing mindset shifts, positive affirmations, and mindfulness practices, individuals with brittle bone disease can empower themselves to overcome adversity and lead fulfilling lives.

Remember that building resilience is not about avoiding challenges or seeking a life free of setbacks. Rather, it is about developing the tools and mindset necessary to navigate these challenges with grace and confidence. With every obstacle faced, you will have the opportunity to grow and become a stronger version of yourself.

So, as you continue on this journey, embrace the power of your thoughts, reinforce positive beliefs through affirmations, and cultivate emotional well-being through mindfulness practices. With these tools, you will not only build resilience and mental strength but also unlock the potential within yourself to live a life of empowerment and fulfillment.

Keep pushing forward, and know that you have the inner strength to overcome anything that comes your way. You are resilient, and you have the power to demystify brittle bone disease and live your best life.

Seeking Professional Help

It can be challenging to emotionally handle any chronic ailment, especially Brittle Bone Disease. Bone fractures are a common occurrence for those who have this illness, and they can leave them feeling sad, angry, frustrated, or even lonely. It can be quite challenging to manage these emotions on one's own, thus receiving professional guidance is highly encouraged.

Psychotherapy and counselling are two therapeutic techniques that can be very beneficial in helping patients deal with the emotional challenges brought on by Brittle Bone Disease. For psychotherapy, also known as talk therapy, a certified therapist who focuses on helping people improve their mental health and general well-being is necessary. In therapy sessions, patients can explore their emotions, identify useful coping strategies, and develop resilience to better manage the ups and downs of life with brittle bone disease.

Counseling programmes can provide specialised support and guidance tailored to the unique challenges caused by brittle bone disease. The therapist can help patients and their loved ones cope with stress and worry, comprehend the emotional implications of the condition, and navigate the complex healthcare system. Counseling can help treat any psychological concerns that may arise, such as depression, anxiety disorders, or body image issues, which are common among persons with chronic illnesses.

Support groups are yet another helpful resource for those with brittle bone disease. These organisations foster a sense of belonging and empathy since their members have gone through similar hardships. Connecting with people who are aware of the condition's physical and mental impacts can be immensely calming and reassuring. Members of support groups can express their emotions freely, get insight from others' experiences, and pick up practical coping skills from those who have successfully managed the emotional effects of having brittle bone disease.

In addition to therapy and support groups, there are several counselling programmes available, each specifically tailored to the requirements of people with Brittle Bone Disease. One such service is genetic counselling. Genetic counselling can be helpful for patients and their families if they wish to understand more about the condition's genetics, think about family planning options, or just have any worries or questions regarding how Brittle Bone Disease is inherited genetically. This therapy may be particularly beneficial for people who wish to start a family or are concerned about passing the problem on to future generations.

For the psychological impacts of brittle bone disease, individuals must take the initiative to seek professional help. Participating in treatment, joining support groups, and participating in counselling can all significantly improve one's quality of life. But it's crucial to get the best specialist to match your goals. Finding experienced therapists who specialise in problems associated with disabilities or long-term illnesses is essential because they will have the expertise and understanding necessary to provide proper support.

When seeking professional assistance, it is crucial to keep in mind interdisciplinary approaches that incorporate a range of healthcare providers. I firmly believe in the importance of collaboration and teamwork as a supporter of holistic medicine. Combining the expertise of therapists, psychologists, nutritionists, and other medical specialists can provide patients with brittle bone disease with comprehensive support. Collaborative consultations can help address the physical, mental, and lifestyle aspects of living with the condition in order to reach an integrated view on well-being.

Getting professional help is essential for managing the psychological impacts of brittle bone disease, to sum up. Therapy options, support groups, and counselling services can all be very beneficial for persons managing the emotional problems that come with living with this condition. Always remember that seeking professional help is a courageous step toward reclaiming control over your emotional wellbeing rather than a sign of weakness. Attending therapy sessions, taking part in support groups, and obtaining counselling services can help people with brittle bone disease develop effective coping skills, find support and understanding, and finally lead fulfilling lives despite the challenges they may face..

Cultivating Supportive Relationships

Humans are social creatures with a social and communal wiring. When we feel that people are seeing, hearing, and getting us, we thrive. This is especially true when dealing with obstacles or trying situations, like the daily struggles brought on by brittle bone disease. By cultivating supportive connections, we not only improve our mental health but also gain the essential skills need to deal with life's ups and downs.

Realizing the value of vulnerability is the first step in developing supportive connections. Although sharing our troubles with others can be intimidating, it is only through being vulnerable that genuine connections can be made. Vulnerability makes room for genuine empathy and understanding by letting people see us for who we really are, warts and all. By accepting vulnerability, we encourage other people to do the same and foster an atmosphere that is conducive to direct and frank conversation.

After accepting our vulnerability, the next step is to actively look for people who will be encouraging and sympathetic. While toxic connections can have the opposite effect, healthy relationships have a significant impact on our emotional wellbeing. Being around by positive and compassionate people makes us feel supported and validated in our battle against brittle bone disease. These people could be relatives, close friends, members of support networks, or even medical experts with expertise in the condition.

But creating a support system takes more than just surrounding ourselves with helpful people; it also entails returning the favour. Relationships that are mutually helpful require us to be there for one another when they are in need as well. Being there for others helps us build stronger relationships and gives our own life a sense of direction and meaning.

Active listening is a proven method for fostering helpful connections. It is crucial to give our whole focus and pay close attention to what others are saying when conversing with family, friends, or members of a support group. This entails putting down outside distractions, such smartphones or other obligations, and concentrating entirely on the person in front of us. By actively listening, we can better understand others and show them that their opinions and feelings matter.

Empathy training is essential in building supportive connections in addition to active listening. Empathy entails putting oneself in another person's situation and comprehending their thoughts and feelings. It necessitates setting aside our own biases and preconceptions in order to fully feel and relate to the experiences of others. By empathising with others, we promote an atmosphere of compassion and understanding, which is crucial for developing helpful connections.

It's critical to be aware of our own needs and boundaries if we want to further build our support systems. Giving and receiving help are both a part of developing supportive relationships, but it's important to avoid exhausting ourselves and putting our own needs last. Recognizing our limitations and establishing boundaries helps us to maintain our energy levels as well as our ability to be present and helpful for others in the long run.

It is equally vital to develop a positive relationship with oneself in addition to interactions with others. Self-compassion and self-care are crucial for fostering resilience and emotional well-being. It is possible for us to present as our best selves in our interactions with others when we take the time to look after our own physical, mental, and emotional health. This can involve actions like developing awareness, taking part in joyful pursuits, obtaining therapy or counselling, and placing a high priority on getting enough rest and relaxation.

Last but not least, it is critical to keep in mind that developing supportive connections requires time and work. Strong support networks are not formed overnight, just as Rome wasn't. It is a continuous process that calls for constant investment and dedication.

It is crucial to constantly remind ourselves of the importance and influence of supporting relationships in fostering emotional well-being, especially at times when we may feel dejected or alone.

Developing and maintaining supportive relationships is crucial for fostering emotional well-being in people with brittle bone disease. We may build a solid support system that enables us to face life's obstacles with resilience and strength by embracing vulnerability, seeking out supportive people, engaging in active listening and empathy, setting boundaries, and placing a high priority on self-care. Keep in mind that you are not alone on this road, and by developing positive relationships, you can discover the compassion and understanding you need on an emotional level..

Chapter 6: Empowering Independence and Accessibility

Home Modifications for Accessibility

As a physician and health and wellness coach, I have seen firsthand the difficulties that people with Brittle Bone Disease have. Their movement and independence may be significantly restricted by the brittleness of their bones and propensity for fractures. Making their homes a secure and accessible space is essential because of this..

Bathrooms: Due to the slick surfaces and small confines, the bathroom can be dangerous for people with brittle bone disease. Several changes can be done to reduce these hazards.

Installing grab bars next to the toilet, in the shower, and next to the bathtub is crucial first and foremost. When getting in and out of the shower or transferring to and from the toilet, these bars offer stability and support. It is essential to check that these bars are firmly fastened to the wall, strong enough to support the person's weight, and set up at a convenient height.

For people with restricted mobility, shower chairs or benches can be just as helpful as grab bars. This lowers their danger of falling because they can sit while taking a shower. Shower chairs should have stable backrests and non-slip feet to offer support and stability.

Consider constructing a higher toilet seat to further improve accessibility in the restroom, which can make it simpler for people with Brittle Bone Disease to sit down and stand up. A handheld showerhead can also be helpful for people with mobility issues because it enables them to easily adjust the direction and flow of water while sitting..

Bedrooms: People with Brittle Bone Disease frequently spend a lot of time in their bedrooms. It ought to be cosy, secure, and convenient.

The height of the bed is one of the most crucial alterations to take into account. Individuals may find it simpler to freely climb into and out of bed if the bed height is lowered. This can be accomplished by utilising a low-profile bed frame or by placing a mattress on the floor without a box spring. In order to avoid any accidents, it is essential to make sure the bed is secure and firm.

Another essential component of a secure and accessible bedroom is appropriate lighting. Brittle Bone Disease patients can see their surroundings clearly with the aid of adequate lighting, which lowers their risk of accidents and falls. Consider employing motion sensor lights to illuminate the path to the restroom or other locations at night in addition to installing bright, adjustable lighting fixtures.

To enhance accessibility, furniture arrangement should be carefully planned. Make sure there is sufficient room to move a wheelchair or other mobility aids without strain. Eliminate any debris or obstructions that can obstruct movement.

Living Spaces: It's crucial to make adjustments in other rooms of the house outside the toilet and bedroom to improve accessibility and foster independence.

Make sure that every doorway and walkway is broad enough to fit a wheelchair or other mobility aid before anything else. For ease accessibility, a minimum entryway width of 32 inches is advised. Take out any extra rugs or carpets that could be a trip hazard.

People with restricted mobility might benefit immensely from railings installed along steps. These handrails must to be firmly installed and offer assistance on both sides of the staircase. Non-slip stair treads can be added to increase security and lower the chance of accidents.

The location of electrical outlets and light switches should also be taken into account. These can be placed at a lower height to make them more reachable for people who find it difficult to comfortably visit higher places. Installing voice-activated lighting and thermostats that can be operated without making physical touch is another worthwhile consideration.

To improve accessibility and encourage independence, changes might be done in the kitchen. Pull-out shelves or drawers can improve visibility and access to stored things, and lowering counters and cabinets might make them easier to reach. Lever-style handles can be added to cabinet doors and faucets to make them simpler for those with weak hands to use.

Finally, it's critical to develop an emergency plan and make sure that everyone in the household is aware of it. This involves having easy access to the appropriate medical supplies, clear instructions for emergency responders, and accessible exits.

Conclusion:

Individuals with Brittle Bone Disease can feel more independent, secure, and comfortable by adopting certain accessibility-related home adjustments. These modifications to the bathroom, bedroom, and other living areas can greatly enhance their quality of life and make it easier for them to move around their houses. To guarantee that these alterations are tailored to each person's needs and requirements, it is crucial to engage with healthcare professionals, contractors, and accessibility specialists..

Assistive Technology for Independence

Mobility Aids:

Mobility can frequently be difficult for those who have Brittle Bone Disease because of the fragility and fracture-proneness of their bones. Different mobility tools can significantly increase independence and make it easier for people with Brittle Bone Disease to move about their environment. I'll go over a few of the most popular mobility aids here:

1. Wheelchairs: A crucial piece of assistive technology for people with limited mobility is a wheelchair. There are various sorts of wheelchairs available, including those that the user pushes themselves or those that are driven by a motor. The individual's personal needs and level of mobility will determine the wheelchair that is best for them.

2. Scooters: For those with stronger upper body stability and strength, scooters offer an alternative to wheelchairs. These mobility aids are very helpful for people who just need a little support but still need help travelling farther or participating in outdoor activities.

3. Walkers: Patients with Brittle Bone Disease who have some degree of mobility and strength in their legs frequently utilise walkers, also known as Zimmer frames. Walkers offer support and stability during walking, reducing the risk of falls and fractures.

4. Crutches: People with Brittle Bone Disease who can support themselves while walking but lack the upper body strength frequently need crutches. They provide extra assistance and help keep things balanced.

Communication Devices:

For people with Brittle Bone Disease, effective communication is essential because it enables them to express their needs and interact with others. Communication devices can be useful assistive technologies for fostering independence and facilitating meaningful interactions. Here are a few instances of communication devices:

1. Augmentative and Alternative Communication (AAC) Devices: AAC devices are made to help those who have trouble communicating. These gadgets can be as basic as graphic boards or as advanced as speech-generating systems that let users choose and speak certain words or phrases. AAC tools can be customised to a person's unique needs, promoting freedom and assuring successful communication.

2. Computer-based Communication Systems: People with limited mobility can use computer-based communication technologies, such as eye gaze technology or head-controlled devices, to access computers and communicate with others. To translate user inputs into spoken or written language, these systems need specialised software and hardware.

3. Voice Amplifiers: Voice amplifiers are compact, portable devices that improve a user's natural voice to help them be heard in a variety of situations. These tools are especially helpful for those with Brittle Bone Disease who might struggle to project their voice or have weaker vocal muscles.

Adaptive Tools:

People with Brittle Bone Disease can profit from a range of adapted technologies that help with daily tasks and foster independence, in addition to mobility assistance and communication aids. These devices are made to make up for physical constraints, making it simpler for people to carry out tasks that they might find difficult otherwise. Here are a few illustrations of adaptable tools:

1. Adaptive Clothing: Adaptive clothing is created specifically to meet the specific requirements and difficulties of people with reduced mobility. Easy-to-reach zippers, adjustable waistbands, and Velcro closures making it simpler and more comfortable to dress and undress.

2. Assistive Eating Devices: For those with Brittle Bone Disease, assistive eating tools such customised utensils and non-slip plates can considerably improve autonomous eating. The ergonomic design of

these equipment increases stability and control while lowering the possibility of spills or mishaps.

3. Adaptive Tools for Personal Care: For those with limited mobility, assistive gadgets for personal care, such as specialised grooming aids, long-handled brushes, and adaptable shower seats, can make activities like bathing, grooming, and using the restroom more bearable.

4. Environmental Modifications: For those with brittle bone disease, changing the surroundings can dramatically increase freedom and accessibility. Installing grab bars in bathrooms, stairlifts or ramps for improved movement, and altering furniture heights to suit wheelchair or scooter users are a few examples of environmental alterations.

Conclusion:

In order to encourage independence and raise quality of life for people with brittle bone disease, assistive devices are essential. Mobility aids, communication tools, and adaptive equipment all help people be more physically mobile, communicate effectively, and carry out daily duties more easily. Brittle bone disease patients can overcome physical obstacles and lead full lives by integrating these assistive technology into their daily lives.

Accessible Transportation Options

Assess Your Needs

It's important to evaluate your unique demands and requirements before looking into transportation solutions. Think about the following elements:

1. Mobility: Consider your physical prowess and any mobility restrictions. Do you need a wheelchair or other assistive device? Are you able to independently transfer from your wheelchair to a car?

2. Assistance: Ascertain whether you need support while travelling. Do you require assistance using the public transportation system or getting in and out of the car?

3. Medical equipment: Consider any medical supplies or equipment you would need to transport, such as oxygen tanks.

You may reduce your alternatives and choose the best kind of transportation by being aware of your demands..

Choosing a Suitable Vehicle

Choosing a proper vehicle is essential for people with Brittle Bone Disease to guarantee comfort, safety, and accessibility. When choosing a vehicle, take into account the following factors:

1. Wheelchair accessibility: Look for vehicles that are accessible if you require a wheelchair. These automobiles have ramps, lifts, and other adaptations that make wheelchair entry and egress simple.

2. Height and seating: Make sure there is enough height and space in the car for people with Brittle Bone Disease. Seek out cars with adjustable seats and lots of room for stretching and adjusting your body in a comfortable manner.

3. Safety features: Give preference to cars with sophisticated safety features like stability control, airbags, and anti-lock brakes. In the case of an accident, these features offer an additional degree of safety.

4. Ease of entry and exit: If you have limited mobility, choose vehicles with large door openings and low step-in heights to make entering and exiting them easier.

Public Transportation Accessibility

Public transportation is another good choice for those with Brittle Bone Disease, even though accessible private vehicles provide convenience, independence, and control. Here are some things to think about before using public transportation:

1. Research local accessibility: Look at your area's public transit options' accessibility. Verify whether wheelchair access ramps or lifts are available on buses, trains, and trams. To make moving around easier, find out if stations and stops have escalators or elevators.

2. Identify accessible routes: Choose a few routes that pass by accessible stations and stops that are close to the places you want to go. Your travel experience can go more smoothly if you plan beforehand and become familiar with accessible routes.

3. Utilize assistive devices: Consider employing assistive devices, such as mobility aids or portable ramps, depending on your needs to make boarding and disembarking public transportation easier.

4. Seek assistance: Ask about additional help or assistance that is offered for people with impairments by contacting customer service departments or public transit authority. For people with mobility issues, several public transportation networks provide customised services or paratransit options.

Resources for Travel Planning

Making your travel arrangements in advance can reduce stress and guarantee a positive experience. Here are some excellent tools to help with travel preparation:

1. Online resources: Investigate the websites and online resources that offer details on accessible transportation options. Look for listings of accessibility features, user ratings, and different transit services..

2. App-based services: Make use of mobile applications that provide accessible transportation options. These apps frequently let you schedule rides, keep track of your travels, and provide details on accessible vehicles.

3. Disability travel agencies: Consider contacting specialised travel businesses that assist people with disabilities. These organisations are skilled and knowledgeable in organising accessible travel experiences, and they may offer direction, specific suggestions, and help in locating the best transportation options.

4. Local disability organizations: Join a local advocacy or support group for people with disabilities. When it comes to accessible transportation choices in your area, they might be able to give resources, advice, or direct knowledge.

By using these tools, you can gain the knowledge and assistance needed to efficiently organise your trip and guarantee a safe and convenient vacation..

In Conclusion,

For people with Brittle Bone Disease to retain their independence and quality of life, accessible transportation is essential. You may move confidently and easily through the world of transportation by determining your needs, selecting an appropriate car, looking into accessible options for public transit, and using tools for travel planning. Always keep in mind that having access to good transportation is essential for your safety, comfort, and freedom to travel to and from any destination..

Education and Employment Accommodations

I have observed how crucial educational and employment accommodations are in ensuring that people with Brittle Bone Disease have equitable opportunity to learn, work, and thrive as a medical practitioner and health and wellness coach. I will share my knowledge and offer a step-by-step tutorial for utilising these technologies in this chapter.

Understanding the Individual's Rights

Understanding the rights of someone with brittle bone disease is the first step in obtaining accommodations for education and work. The Rehabilitation Act of 1973's Section 504 and the Americans with Disabilities Act (ADA) in the United States guarantee legal rights and equal opportunities for people with disabilities.

Individuals with Brittle Bone Disease are entitled to reasonable adjustments in contexts such as schools and workplaces under these laws. By making these adjustments, we hope to level the playing field and remove any obstacles that might get in the way of their success.

Accessing Support Services

Connecting with the relevant support services is crucial after people are aware of their rights. Through the process, these agencies might offer helpful advice and resources. Key support services to take into account include:

1. Disability Services Offices: Disability services offices in educational institutions are experts in offering accommodations to students with disabilities. It is crucial to get in touch with these offices to register for accommodations and submit the required paperwork.

2. Vocational Rehabilitation Services: Individuals with impairments can receive support and help from vocational rehabilitation (VR) programmes in finding and keeping a job.

Assessments, training, career counselling, and referrals to other helpful services are all things that VR organisations can offer.

3. Disability Advocacy Organizations: Many organisations that serve people with disabilities provide resources and support to those who have brittle bone disease. These groups can help people connect with others who share their experiences, advocate for adjustments, and learn their rights.

Identifying Reasonable Accommodations

Finding the precise accommodations that will best help people with Brittle Bone Disease is the next step in the process. Individual needs can be taken into account when making reasonable accommodations, which may include:

1. Assistive Technology: Experiences in education and the workplace can be improved by assistive technology tools and equipment. Software for voice recognition, ergonomic keyboards, and assistive devices are some examples.

2. Flexible Scheduling: People with flexible schedules might modify their work or study hours to suit their own requirements. This can entail modifying the class schedule, offering remote employment opportunities, or setting flexible start and end timings..

3. Physical Modifications: Accessibility can be greatly increased by making physical changes to the working or learning environment. Ramps, railings, automatic doors, and accessible furniture can all be installed as part of this.

4. Note-taking Support: Support for taking notes can be given in a number of ways, such by giving out copies of the lecture notes, employing recording equipment, or using note-taking applications.

5. Emotional Support: It is essential to recognise the emotional toll that having Brittle Bone Disease takes and to offer suitable assistance. Access to counselling services, mindfulness exercises, and peer support groups may be part of this.

Requesting Accommodations and Documentation

Individuals should formally request accommodations from the relevant authorities after determining the necessary accommodations. This can entail providing documents from medical experts outlining the particular need and suggested accommodations. It is essential to make sure that the documentation is thorough and clearly explains the person's condition and functional restrictions.

Collaborating with Educational and Employment Institutions

The person should work closely with educational and employment institutions to build a collaborative and supportive atmosphere after submitting the request for adjustments. To ensure that the accommodations are implemented successfully and that everyone involved is aware of the individual's needs, clear communication is crucial.

Leveraging Advocacy Resources

Utilizing advocacy resources is crucial at every stage of the procedure to guarantee that people with Brittle Bone Disease get the assistance and accommodations to which they are legally entitled. Disability advocacy groups can offer advice on navigating the legal system, engaging in self-advocacy, and making connections with people who share your experiences.

Individuals with Brittle Bone Disease can successfully seek accommodations for school and employment by following this step-by-step manual. It is crucial to keep in mind that everyone's journey will be different, and that the process could call for persistence and patience. However, people who have Brittle Bone Disease can create circumstances that promote their career and personal development if they have the correct information and assistance. Let's examine the advantages of accommodations in education and the workplace and how they can improve the lives of people with brittle bone disease..

Promoting Inclusion and Accessibility in Society

Advocacy Efforts:

In order to raise awareness of Brittle Bone Disease and to advance the rights and welfare of those who are afflicted by it, advocacy is essential. I have seen firsthand the transformative impact of advocacy in removing obstacles and enhancing accessibility in society as a medical practitioner and health and wellness coach. We may bring about significant changes in a number of elements of the lives of people with Brittle Bone Disease by actively lobbying on their behalf. Access to public spaces, healthcare, education, and work are all included in this.

The goal of advocacy work can be achieved in a variety of ways, from educating the public through educational campaigns to advocating legislation that upholds the rights of people with disabilities. We may raise our voices and have a long-lasting impact by working with patient advocacy groups, doctors, and members of the community. Policy improvements and better inclusion for people with Brittle Bone Disease may result from talks being started at the local, national, and worldwide levels.

Policy Changes:

To ensure that people with Brittle Bone Disease can fully participate in society, policy adjustments are necessary. It is imperative to promote laws that give public accessibility a high priority in areas like transportation, education, employment, and healthcare. By doing this, we can get rid of the physical and interpersonal obstacles that prevent people with this disease from integrating.

The application of inclusive design principles in infrastructure is one illustration of a policy reform that can significantly help people with Brittle Bone Disease. We can build surroundings that are accessible to everyone by taking their needs into account at the planning stage. This can entail building ramps, elevators, and doors with bigger openings to accommodate wheelchairs and other mobility devices. Policies can also be established to guarantee that accessible elements like wheelchair ramps and audiovisual announcements are included in public transportation systems.

Policies should be put in place in the educational sector to give people with Brittle Bone Disease equal access to high-quality education. In order to support children with disabilities, this may entail creating tailored education plans, providing aids and technology, and educating instructors and staff. We can enable people with Brittle Bone Disease to realise their full potential and make a positive contribution to society by ensuring that education is inclusive.

Another major area where policy reforms are required is employment. Employability chances for people with impairments, especially those with Brittle Bone Disease, might be hampered by discrimination and inaccessibility. Promoting laws that support accessible hiring procedures, reasonable modifications, and workplace accessibility can level the playing field and help people with this condition find fulfilling work..

Community Involvement:

Promoting inclusion and accessibility for people with Brittle Bone Disease starts with community involvement. We can build circumstances where these people can flourish by encouraging a sense of acceptance and belonging. Communities are essential in providing resources, understanding, and support to people with disabilities.

Creating social networks and support groups exclusively for people with Brittle Bone Disease and their families is one method to promote community involvement. These communities can provide a forum for experience sharing, emotional support, and the exchange of useful information. Additionally, inclusive events and activities that cater to people with disabilities should be encouraged by community organisations. We can foster a sense of openness and dismantle social barriers by including everyone.

Public education and awareness campaigns can help debunk myths and advance knowledge of the condition known as brittle bone disease. We may promote empathy and acceptance by educating members of the community about the difficulties faced by people with this illness. This can be accomplished by holding workshops, lectures, and public awareness campaigns that promote inclusive behaviour and raise awareness about Brittle Bone Disease.

In conclusion, advancing accessibility and inclusion for people with Brittle Bone Disease in society calls for coordinated initiatives from numerous stakeholders. The creation of a more inclusive and accessible world requires community involvement, policy changes, and advocacy. Together, we can remove obstacles, give people with this condition more power, and make sure they have access to the same opportunities as everyone else. We can effectively demystify brittle bone disease and enhance the lives of those who have it through these combined efforts.

Chapter 7: Living a Fulfilling Life With Brittle Bone Disease

Pursuing Personal Goals and Dreams

I have seen many people with Brittle Bone Disease do incredible things throughout my work as a medical practitioner and health and wellness consultant. Their experiences have served as a monument to the perseverance and brilliance of the human spirit. I want to share a few of these uplifting success stories with you in this part, along with some helpful advice so you can realise your own ambitions.

Let me begin by telling you Sarah's tale. Sarah was diagnosed with brittle bone disease when she was a little girl. Sarah had always wanted to be a ballerina, but her health issues made that seem like an impossibility. Sarah started to pursue her goal, nonetheless, thanks to her unyielding dedication and the help of her family and medical staff. She carefully collaborated with a physical therapist who created a specific workout regimen that prioritised increasing flexibility and strength while lowering the risk of fractures. Additionally, Sarah received instruction from an accomplished ballet teacher who assisted her in modifying conventional ballet techniques to fit her physical constraints.

Sarah's journey was not simple, but she did not let her illness to define who she was. She put in endless practise, always pushing herself to the edge. She could finally see improvement. She developed a grace and elegance that astounded her audience as her movements got more fluid, her balance improved, and she became more graceful. Sarah's tale serves as a powerful illustration of what is achievable if you are persistent and never give up on your goals.

How can you use Sarah's narrative to improve your own life, then? Here are some helpful pointers to assist you in achieving your individual objectives and aspirations:

1. Set Clear Goals: To begin, decide what it is you really want to accomplish. Be explicit and divide your objectives into more

achievable, smaller steps. A roadmap that will direct you on your trip can be made by having a clear vision of what you want to achieve.

2. Gather Support: Embrace a group of professionals, close friends, and members of your family who have faith in you and your talents. Find people who can support and guide you as you work toward your objectives. Medical experts who are familiar with your illness and can assist you in creating a strategy that puts your health and safety first should be on this team.

3. Adapt and Modify: Even though you have physical restrictions, you can still accomplish your goals. Be willing to adjust and change your strategy to fit your condition. This can entail looking for different ways to accomplish your objectives or making changes to better suit your unique requirements.

4. Focus on Strengths: Recognizing and celebrating your talents is just as crucial as understanding and accepting your limitations. Use your strengths to your advantage by identifying the abilities, talents, and characteristics that you possess. You may maximise your chance of success by using your strengths.

5. Take Care of Yourself: It takes a strong commitment to self-care to manage a chronic ailment. Adopt healthy lifestyle practises that put your physical, emotional, and mental wellness first. This can be getting regular exercise into your schedule, eating healthily, doing things to relieve stress, and getting therapy or counselling as needed.

6. Practice Resilience: Setbacks are frequently a part of any road towards reaching your goals because life is full of ups and downs. To overcome disappointments and setbacks, resilience development is essential. Develop a positive outlook, see obstacles as chances for development, and draw wisdom from your experiences.

Just keep in mind that while the path to realising your personal aspirations may not always be straightforward, it is always worthwhile. You shouldn't let the difficulties brought on by brittle bone disease stop you from pursuing your passions. You can overcome every challenge that comes your way if you have the proper attitude, the appropriate help, and the right commitment.

In conclusion, I hope that this chapter has motivated you to strive for your personal ambitions, despite any obstacles that Brittle Bone Disease may present. Take inspiration from others who have triumphed despite the obstacles, and use the helpful advice given to forge your own course to success. Keep in mind that you are capable of greatness and that your aspirations are attainable. Accept where you are going and keep your priorities in focus..

Exploring Adaptive Hobbies and Recreation

This section examines the range of adapted pastimes and leisure pursuits available to people with brittle bone disease. It encourages users to find new passions by providing advice, resources, and success stories.

I have worked directly with people with Brittle Bone Disease to assist them lead meaningful lives despite their physical limitations as a clinician and health coach. Participating in adapted hobbies and leisure activities is one thing that frequently gives these people a great deal of joy and satisfaction. We will examine the many alternatives in this chapter, offering in-depth analysis and suggestions for readers wishing to discover new interests.

The Importance of Adaptive Hobbies and Recreation

Living with brittle bone disease can be difficult on a physical and psychological level. Feelings of dissatisfaction and solitude might result from the ongoing possibility of fractures and restricted mobility. Recreational activities that are adaptive not only offer a much-needed break from these challenges but also foster a sense of empowerment and accomplishment.

Adaptive pastimes and leisure pursuits are made specifically to assist people with physical limitations. People with Brittle Bone Disease can engage in these activities to follow their passions and interests, which gives them a feeling of purpose and fulfilment. Adaptive choices enable people with Brittle Bone Disease to enjoy the excitement and satisfaction that comes from participating in these activities, whether it's painting, playing an instrument, or playing sports..

Adaptive Hobbies and Recreational Activities

1. **Creative Pursuits:**

- *Painting and Drawing:* The best way for people with Brittle Bone Disease to express their creativity is through art. Adaptive art supplies like easel attachments and paintbrush holders can make the process simpler and more fun..
   - *Sculpting and Pottery:* Beautiful sculptures made of clay can be relaxing and rewarding to work on. People with poor dexterity may be able to experiment with this art form thanks to adaptive gear like hand braces and altered pottery wheels.
   - *Writing and Poetry:* For those with Brittle Bone Disease, writing out their thoughts and feelings can be cathartic. For those with poor hand function, typing assistance and speech-to-text software can make the task easier.
   2. **Music and Performance:**
   - *Instrumental Music:* Not only is playing an instrument a method to express oneself, but it also enhances cognitive function and reduces stress. Adaptive instruments, like guitar neck modifications and piano key extensions, allow people with Brittle Bone Disease to enjoy music.
   - *Singing and Vocal Performance:* Singing and vocal performance can be an excellent way for people with limited hand use to interact with music. Taking voice lessons or joining a choir can give one a sense of success and community.
   - *Dance and Movement:* Dance lessons and programmes for people with physical limitations, such as Brittle Bone Disease, are available. These exercises have a strong emphasis on individual expression, creativity, and movement.
   3. **Sports and Recreation:**
   - *Wheelchair Basketball:* With the help of this adaptive sport, people with mobility issues can experience the thrill of competitive basketball. Participants can improve their skills and compete at different levels thanks to modified wheelchairs and court adaptations..

- *Archery:* With the use of adaptive gear like arm braces and adapted bows, people with Brittle Bone Disease can participate in archery, an activity that calls on accuracy and concentration. Participants can enhance their hand-eye coordination and self-confidence by participating in archery.

- *Swimming:* Swimming is a great sport for those with Brittle Bone Disease since water-based activities are easy on the bones and joints. Adaptive swimwear and flotation aids offer assistance and protection, enabling people to enjoy the water without worrying about getting hurt.

4. **Outdoor and Adventure Activities:**

- *Nature Photography:* For someone with restricted mobility, taking photographs of nature's beauty can be a pleasant hobby. Now that smartphones and affordable camera gear are available, everyone can delve into the realm of photography.

- *Gardening:* For people with brittle bone disease, gardening and caring for plants can be therapeutic and enjoyable activities. For people with physical disabilities, gardening is more accessible thanks to raised beds, adjustable tools, and assistive technologies.

- *Camping and Hiking:* A sense of adventure and a connection with nature can be found through camping and hiking. People with Brittle Bone Disease can engage in these activities safely and pleasantly thanks to adaptive camping equipment and open-access routes.

Resources and Testimonials:

There are numerous resources available to assist people with Brittle Bone Disease in exploring adaptive hobbies and leisure pursuits in addition to the recommendations made above. Finding adapted programmes and making connections with like-minded people is made easier with the help of local community centres, organisations for people with disabilities, and online resources.

Testimonials from people who have taken up adapted hobbies and leisure pursuits can also offer insightful information and motivation.

Hearing about people who overcame physical obstacles to follow their ambitions might serve as a motivational reminder that everything is possible with tenacity and flexibility..

In Conclusion,

The world of adaptable pastimes and leisure pursuits for people with brittle bone disease has been examined in this chapter. These pursuits help people feel more content and fulfilled, which improves their overall wellbeing. Brittle bone disease patients can find new passions and create a life that is full of creativity, accomplishment, and joy by embracing adaptive options and looking for resources and support.

Advocacy and Making a Difference

As a physician and wellness coach, advocacy has always been at the heart of my work. It is important to recognise the special needs and problems faced by people with Brittle Bone Disease and endeavour to build an inclusive society for them, rather than only treating the physical symptoms and offering medical solutions.

The first step in creating change is raising awareness. Many people are still ignorant of the effects that Brittle Bone Disease has on both sufferers and their families. We can make sure that more people are aware of the difficulties faced by folks with this condition by raising awareness through various channels such public campaigns, social media, and community activities.

It's critical to have a thorough awareness of Brittle Bone Disease and all of its facets in order to effectively advocate for people who suffer from it. This includes understanding the psychological and social effects of having Brittle Bone Disease, as well as the medical components of the condition, ongoing research, and accessible treatment options. With this information, we are better able to express to decision-makers, medical experts, and the general public the needs and worries of people who have Brittle Bone Disease.

An further essential component of lobbying is funding for research. The more money we put into research, the better positioned we are to comprehend the underlying factors causing Brittle Bone Disease, create efficient therapies, and enhance the lives of those who are afflicted. We must work together as the medical community to promote funding for studies on Brittle Bone Disease and to support research projects.

Promoting inclusion is vital for improving the lives of people with Brittle Bone Disease in addition to increasing awareness and funding research. This entails developing accessible and adaptive surroundings and communities for their requirements. It entails speaking out for equality in employment, education, and involvement in society as well as dispelling any prejudices or biases that could exist in society.

I have seen firsthand how activism can improve the lives of people with brittle bone disease as a health and fitness coach. By standing up for their needs, we can provide them the tools they need to live successful lives and get through whatever obstacles they may encounter. This entails educating them about the resources that are out there, putting them in touch with social networks, and assisting them in developing self-advocacy abilities.

Amplifying those with Brittle Bone Disease's voices is one of the most effective strategies to fight for their rights. Too frequently, their viewpoints and experiences are obscured or disregarded. We can reduce the distance between people with this ailment and the general public by aggressively searching out their tales and disseminating them. This can dispel myths and promote empathy and comprehension.

Each and every one of us may participate in advocacy; it is not just for experts and healthcare workers. We all have the capacity to change things, whether it's by volunteering, giving to organisations that support research into Brittle Bone Disease, or just raising awareness of the issue among ourselves and others. It's crucial to keep in mind that even seemingly insignificant actions can make a big difference in the lives of people who suffer from Brittle Bone Disease.

In conclusion, improving the lives of people with Brittle Bone Disease requires advocating and making a difference. We can build a society that recognises, values, and empowers persons with this disease by increasing awareness, funding research, and fostering inclusivity. It is our duty as healthcare professionals to set an example and fight for the interests and rights of people with brittle bone disease. Without regard to a person's health, we can work together to build a world where everyone has equal possibilities.

Celebrating Achievements and Milestones

Brittle bone disease can make daily life difficult. It might frequently seem like an uphill struggle, with many setbacks and barriers in the way. But it's important to keep in mind that every little triumph should be honoured. Every success, no matter how small it may appear, is a testimonial to one's tenacity and perseverance, whether it be taking a few steps without help or realising a particular objective.

Celebrating successes is a great way to increase drive and self-confidence. It's not just about enjoying the moment. By praising our accomplishments, we strengthen the idea that we are capable of more. We prove to ourselves that we are capable of overcoming the challenges presented by Brittle Bone Disease and that our efforts are not in vain.

Setting realistic goals is one of the most important components of celebrating accomplishments. Setting high standards that are practically impossible to achieve can be demoralising. Instead, it's crucial to divide bigger objectives into more achievable stages. For instance, start by taking a stroll around the neighbourhood and gradually increase the distance over time rather than setting out to climb a mountain. We boost our chances of success by setting attainable goals, which provides us more reasons to rejoice.

Recognizing the effort required to reach these milestones is also essential. Living with brittle bone disease frequently calls for more commitment and tenacity. It entails receiving medical care, following a certain diet, and making a number of lifestyle adjustments. We give ourselves the credit we deserve by acknowledging the effort put out in managing the condition.

Celebrating successes and significant anniversaries shouldn't be done alone. It is essential to have a network of people at our sides who can celebrate with us and provide us support when we need it. Family, close friends, medical experts, or even online groups of people with similar experiences might be a part of this support system. Sharing our successes with others not only increases the happiness but also fosters a sense of connection and belonging.

It is crucial to recognise milestones within the larger community affected by Brittle Bone Disease in addition to personal accomplishments. Research breakthroughs, better available treatments, or campaigns to increase public awareness of the ailment could all be considered among these milestones. By celebrating these accomplishments, we promote unity and group progress.

The act of taking pleasure in our achievements can transform us. It enables us to focus on the possibilities rather than the constraints that Brittle Bone Disease can place on our life. It is beneficial to change our perspective from one of hopelessness and annoyance to one of fortitude and thankfulness. It serves as a reminder that despite difficulties, there is always cause for celebration.

I'll offer helpful tactics and resources throughout this section to support people with Brittle Bone Disease in marking their victories and anniversaries. These tactics will cover a range of topics, such as mental, emotional, and physical health. They will be founded on a holistic view of healthcare, taking into account the fact that true wellness goes beyond the physical.

I'll go into detail on the value of self-care habits and how they may help us feel successful and content. Readers are urged to investigate pursuits that make them happy and feel accomplished, from embracing relaxing methods like meditation and deep breathing exercises to indulging in creative outlets like art or writing.

In this chapter, nutrition will also be an important subject. For people with Brittle Bone Disease, a balanced diet can significantly promote overall health and wellbeing. Readers will be able to celebrate the accomplishments of keeping a balanced diet and enjoying greater vigour by concentrating on nutrient-dense foods that support bone health and comprehending how certain dietary choices might effect their condition.

I will also go over the significance of mental and emotional health because Brittle Bone Disease frequently has a negative impact on these areas of one's life. By using methods like cognitive-behavioral therapy, gratitude exercises, and mindfulness techniques, people can learn to enjoy the present moment and become resilient in the face of difficulties.

In the end, this section will act as a guide to assist people with Brittle Bone Disease in celebrating their accomplishments and milestones, regardless of how big or small. Readers will be given the tools they need to live full lives despite the difficulties caused by their condition by highlighting the value of celebrating victories, setting attainable objectives, and developing a support network..

Embracing Positivity and Gratitude

Let's first comprehend the importance of these two crucial components in our lives before we dig further into the methods for adopting positivity and thankfulness. Positive thinking and thankfulness can have a significant impact on our physical and mental health, as demonstrated by several scientific studies.

Emmons and McCullough's 2003 study, which was published in the Journal of Personality and Social Psychology, reveals that thankfulness is essential for lowering stress and depressive symptoms. It encourages deeper sleep, strengthens the immune system, and improves general psychological wellness. Positive feelings have even been shown to boost longevity and life happiness, according to research.

Beyond the research investigations, allow me to share with you a personal encounter. I became aware of the power of optimism and appreciation at a young age because they were engrained in my family's daily life. My father, who is also a physician, has always emphasised the value of finding happiness in the little things and being appreciative of what we have.

This frame of mind ultimately inspired me to concentrate on promoting holistic healthcare and wellbeing by assisting me in navigating the difficulties of my own medical journey. And now, it is my goal to share this knowledge with you, my dear readers, so that you can also benefit from the positive and gratifying influence in your own lives.

So let's get started with some doable strategies for embracing optimism and gratitude:

1. Practice Mindfulness: Being completely present in the present and observing our thoughts and sensations without passing judgement on them are the practises of mindfulness. Daily mindfulness practise helps us recognise our negative thought patterns and replace them

with constructive ones. This can aid in mental adjustment and the development of a more upbeat attitude on life.

2. Keep a Gratitude Journal: Create a thankfulness diary and make it a habit of listing a few things each day that you are thankful for. It might be as straightforward as a warm cup of tea or a call from a close friend. You can teach your mind to look for and appreciate the excellent in every circumstance by keeping your attention on the positives.

3. Surround Yourself with Positivity: Whether it be through books, podcasts, or people in your life, surround yourself with uplifting influences. Look for motivational and inspirational sources that will improve your spirits and help you maintain a good outlook. Carefully consider the company you join because negativity might spread.

4. Practice Positive Self-Talk: Be aware of your inner conversation and replace unfavourable statements with supportive ones. Remind yourself of your qualities, accomplishments, and advancements. Celebrate your minor accomplishments and treat yourself with kindness and respect.

5. Find Joy in Simple Pleasures: Develop awe for the small things in life and an appreciation for them. Take the time to appreciate these moments and find gratitude in the here and now, whether it's a stunning sunset, a soft blanket, or a tasty meal.

Along with these strategies, it's important to understand that practising thankfulness and positivity might be difficult on occasion. This is typical, and it's vital to keep in mind that it's appropriate to experience sadness occasionally. Give yourself the time and space to process these feelings while allowing yourself to fully enjoy them.

But even in the most trying circumstances, there is always cause for optimism and appreciation. It might be a loved one's encouragement, a stranger's smile, or the resiliency you have developed as a result of your experiences. Keep these feelings of thankfulness close at hand and use them to help you return to a good frame of mind.

In summary, cultivating optimism and thankfulness involves turning our attention away from the difficulties we confront in favour of the gifts all around us. It is about finding comfort and strength in the little successes and letting the force of positivity push us up. Despite the challenges that Brittle Bone Disease may provide, we may create a fulfilling life by developing a grateful attitude and practising appreciation.

Therefore, I implore you, my dear readers, to begin this road of embracing positivity and thankfulness with an open heart and mind. Accept the ability you have to create your own reality, and let appreciation serve as your compass even in the most difficult circumstances. Always keep in mind that there are opportunities for development, healing, and joy even in the face of adversity every day..

Chapter 8: Insights From Brittle Bone Disease Patients

Stories of Resilience and Overcoming Challenges

Emily's Story:

Let me introduce you to Emily, a fantastic young lady who has triumphed despite her fragile bones and beaten the odds. Osteogenesis imperfecta, a disorder that made Emily's bones exceedingly brittle and prone to fractures, was identified in her at a young age. While many people would have let their illness dictate and restrict their life, Emily had different ideas.

Emily experienced multiple fractured bones as a child, numerous surgeries, and unending hospital stays. Emily made the decision to see these situations as nothing more than obstacles to get beyond, even though they could have made her feel hopeless and dejected. She worked tirelessly toward her goal of becoming a professional dancer.

The road Emily took to becoming a dancer wasn't simple. Her brittle bones required her to change how she moved and how she used certain techniques. She developed secure and efficient training plans in close collaboration with her medical staff, which also included orthopaedic doctors and physical therapists. She beat all odds and gained admission to a prominent dancing school via sheer resolve.

Emily was able to prove to herself and others that her disability did not define her thanks to dance, which also gave her a physical release and a platform for self-expression. She shared her tale via her performances, encouraging many others to embrace their own resiliency and overcome obstacles.

Adam's Story:

Let me now tell you about Adam's inspiring path, a young man who has changed both his own life and the lives of those affected by brittle bone disease. Adam was born with the illness, and during his youth, he underwent numerous medical procedures and fractures, as is common for children with Osteogenesis Imperfecta.

However, Adam's resilience would really be put to the test when he was a teenager. His severe spinal anomalies required a number of procedures, including the insertion of metal rods to strengthen his brittle bones. Although recovering from these operations was difficult and painful, Adam didn't let it get to him.

Adam started a nonprofit organisation because he was determined to make a difference and build a network of support for others dealing with same difficulties. Through this group, he promoted knowledge of Brittle Bone Disease and offered assistance to those with the ailment as well as their families.

Adam's group developed into a glimmer of hope for individuals who were feeling helpless and overtaken by their situation. He was all too aware of the frustration and isolation that frequently accompany living with brittle bone disease due to his personal experiences. Adam was steadfastly determined to make sure that nobody other had to go through those challenges alone.

His organisation provided a wide range of help services, such as instructional materials, counselling, peer support groups, and even financial aid for medical costs. Adam made sure that others have the resources and support system they required to deal with the difficulties of living with brittle bone disease through these efforts..

Conclusion:

These inspirational tales of resiliency and triumph against hardship are proof of the resilience of the human spirit. Adam and Emily refused to allow their illness limit or define them. They not only overcome their own obstacles thanks to their unyielding tenacity, but they also turned into symbols of inspiration and hope for others.

Their experiences serve as a reminder that resilience is a quality that all of us possess, not just a select few. We may overcome the difficulties we encounter by finding our own inner strength, accepting our frailties, and asking for help from others.

It is normal to feel overpowered and defeated when faced with difficulty. But these tales demonstrate that there is light even in the most hopeless situations. By sharing their own experiences, Emily and Adam hope to inspire everyone to find their own routes to resilience and to remember that difficulties do not define who we are; rather, they only serve to bolster our spirit..

Perspectives on Living With Brittle Bone Disease

Chapter 5: Perspectives on Living with Brittle Bone Disease

Living with brittle bone disease can provide a variety of physical and emotional difficulties. We will hear from those who have personally dealt with this disease and are prepared to share their experiences, ideas, and advice in this chapter. Their viewpoints will offer priceless insights into the particular struggles and day-to-day struggles faced by people with Brittle Bone Disease.

1. Sarah's Journey: Finding Strength Amidst Fragility

A 35-year-old lady named Sarah discusses her experience coping with Brittle Bone Disease and the methods she uses to maintain both her physical and psychological health. Due to an uncommon bone condition she was born with, Sarah fractured a lot as a child. She remembers her family's unshakable conviction in her strength and how it helped her develop resilience with fondness.

Sarah still encounters difficulties because of her handicap as an adult. She has however come to understand the value of self-care methods for stress management and mindset maintenance. Sarah stresses the value of giving attention to mental health while navigating the physical constraints brought on by Brittle Bone Disease, whether through regular mindfulness practises or participating in hobbies that make her happy.

2. Mark's Advice: Embracing Adaptability and Independence

The perspective of Mark, a 42-year-old man with brittle bone disease, is provided, along with suggestions for those dealing with similar difficulties. He discusses the value of adaptation in daily life and how he has developed the ability to change his surroundings in order to meet his demands. Mark believes in taking practical measures to promote safety and independence, such as placing grab bars in his bathroom and adopting assistive technology.

Mark discusses how he actively searches out medical specialists who are knowledgeable with Brittle Bone Disease and can offer proper care, emphasising the need of self-advocacy. Mark has been able to retain a high quality of life despite his disability by creating a solid support system and managing his healthcare..

3. Lisa's Reflections: Overcoming Societal Perceptions and Stigmas

The experience of Lisa, a 28-year-old woman with brittle bone disease, in managing cultural preconceptions and stigmas related to disability is shared here. She experienced misinterpretation and discrimination because of her condition beginning in childhood. Lisa emphasises the value of education and awareness in dispelling stereotypes regarding disabilities.

She provides insightful advice on fostering inclusivity and boosting self-confidence. Lisa regularly participates in advocacy work with the goal of removing barriers that people with disabilities confront and fostering a more inclusive society. Lisa inspires people with Brittle Bone Disease to embrace their distinctive talents and not let societal norms dictate their value via her experiences..

4. Mike's Tips: Thriving Through Physical Activity and Support

A 50-year-old man with brittle bone disease named Mike discusses his path to embrace physical activity and the beneficial effects it has had on his general well-being. Despite the fragility of his bones, Mike thinks it's critical to be active in order to preserve muscular strength and stop more BBD issues.

He talks about different low-impact workouts that have benefitted his physical and mental wellbeing, including yoga and swimming. Mike also discusses the critical importance of support from medical experts, family, and friends in his quest to thrive despite having brittle bone disease.

Conclusion:

These perspectives from people with brittle bone disease provide priceless insights into the daily struggles, victories, and coping mechanisms associated with this condition. These people open the door to understanding and compassionate care for patients with Brittle Bone Disease by sharing their experiences, ideas, and recommendations. Their experiences serve as a reminder that having a chronic illness does not necessarily entail leading a life devoid of hope, happiness, and fulfilment. Brittle bone disease sufferers can live happy lives and discover strength in their fragility with the correct assistance, coping mechanisms, and a positive outlook.

Building Support Networks and Community

It can feel lonely to have brittle bone disease. You may be unable to participate in some activities due to the physical restrictions imposed by the disease, and it may be difficult to build relationships with others. But it's important to keep in mind that you're not by yourself. By actively looking for others who can relate to and empathise with your experiences, you can build a network of support that will aid you in overcoming the particular difficulties you face.

I have personally experienced the transforming effect of creating a solid support network during the years that I have worked as a medical doctor and health and wellness coach. By getting in touch with people who have gone through similar things, you might not only find comfort but also obtain essential information and insights that will help you take better control of your condition.

What steps can you take to create a sense of community and a support system? Let's look at some pointers and methods that can support you on this journey:

1. Connect with Local Support Groups: Contact regional groups or organisations that offer support to people with Brittle Bone Disease or other comparable chronic diseases. These organisations frequently plan get-togethers, workshops, and other activities that let you interact with people going through comparable struggles. Participating in these events can foster friendship and provide an opportunity for sharing experiences..

2. Utilize Online Communities: Connecting with people around the world is now simpler than ever thanks to the development of technology. You can communicate with people who are familiar with your path by connecting with them in online communities and forums devoted to brittle bone disease. Join these communities, take part in

the discussions, and gain from the knowledge and perceptions of other participants.

3. Seek Peer Support: Speak with those who have experienced brittle bone disease for a longer period of time. These peers have a plethora of information and useful advice based on their own experiences. You can obtain a wider view on coping mechanisms, therapeutic choices, and daily life approaches by getting in touch with them. Peer support can help reassure you that you are not alone in your troubles and that you can still have a happy life despite the difficulties.

4. Foster Meaningful Relationships: Finding individuals who share your condition does not suffice to form a support network. It also involves developing sincere relationships with people who are interested in you as a person and not just your medical history. Find those who will listen to you, be there for you emotionally, and encourage you on your path. These connections can uplift you, strengthen your fortitude, and give you the inspiration you need to keep going.

5. Engage in Supportive Activities: Participating in activities created especially for people with Brittle Bone Disease can present uncommon chances to interact and create friendships. Look for leisure clubs, art therapy programmes, or adaptive sports teams that serve people with impairments. In addition to fostering a feeling of community, these activities give you the chance to have meaningful experiences that improve your overall well-being.

6. Embrace Virtual Support: Physical distance is no longer a barrier to our ability to connect with others in the modern digital world. For those who are physically isolated or have limited mobility, virtual support networks, such as online video chats or support groups on social media platforms, can be a lifeline. Accept these online spaces as a way to communicate, exchange ideas, and get advice from people in similar situations.

7. Educate Your Loved Ones: Connecting with people who do not just suffer Brittle Bone Disease is an important part of creating a support system. It also includes the people that love and care for you on a daily basis. Inform your loved ones, close friends, and caregivers of the difficulties you are experiencing and the help you need. Help them comprehend how they can support you and act as allies along the way. By encouraging their involvement and empathy, you build a network of support that goes beyond your own neighbourhood.

Please keep in mind that establishing a support system and a sense of community is a dynamic and ever-evolving process. Allowing others into your life requires patience, vulnerability, and hard work. Be receptive to these relationships, enjoy the experiences they bring, and offer assistance in return. You will discover strength, resiliency, and an unfailing support system in establishing and nurturing these relationships, and they will accompany you on your journey through the difficulties of brittle bone disease.

In conclusion, individuals with Brittle Bone Disease must establish solid support systems and a sense of community. You can build a support network that fosters your overall well-being by actively pursuing relationships, participating in activities, and embracing both physical and virtual platforms. Do not forget that you are not travelling alone on this road, my dear readers. As you traverse the path of life with brittle bone disease, reach out, make connections, and let the strength of community to inspire and direct you.

Promoting Awareness and Advocacy

Osteogenesis Imperfecta (OI), often known as brittle bone disease, is a hereditary illness characterised by weak, easily broken bones. People from many walks of life are affected, and those who are diagnosed with the disorder deal with many difficulties on a daily basis. Nevertheless, despite these difficulties, many sufferers with brittle bone disease have demonstrated remarkable fortitude and tenacity in raising awareness and defending their own rights.

One such uplifting tale comes from Sarah, a young person who has battled brittle bone disease her entire life. Sarah has made it her mission to clarify myths and increase awareness of the condition. She launched a blog where she is openly sharing her experiences and giving readers a glimpse into what it's really like to live with brittle bone disease. Sarah discusses the psychological and physical difficulties she encounters on her blog and informs readers about many facets of the illness. In order to enable people with Brittle Bone Disease to take control of their health and well-being, she also stresses the value of self-care and self-advocacy.

Sarah frequently participates in regional and national awareness efforts in addition to blogging. She organises activities that foster awareness and support for folks with the condition in partnership with patient advocacy groups, medical experts, and other people with brittle bone disease. Through their combined efforts, they have been effective in easing access to specialised care for patients with Brittle Bone Disease and raising money for research.

Mark is yet another inspiring person improving the lives of those with brittle bone disease. Early diagnosis of the disease in Mark's son led him to become an advocate for other families dealing with same difficulties. He established a support group exclusively for parents of kids with brittle bone disease, giving them a secure setting in which to share their stories and provide one another with emotional support.

Additionally, Mark arranges educational gatherings and workshops, inviting experts in the field to advise attendees on the most recent approaches to diagnosis and treatment. Through his support group, Mark has built a network of capable parents who can confidently and resolutely handle the complications of brittle bone disease.

To reach a larger audience, many people with Brittle Bone Disease have expanded their advocacy activities into social media platforms. They use social media to connect with others who have had similar situations, share their stories, and offer advice. They make sure their views are heard and the public is informed about brittle bone disease by utilising various hashtags linked to the ailment. These online communities have developed into virtual support networks that give Brittle Bone Disease patients and their loved ones a sense of community and access to a wealth of knowledge and resources.

Along with individual activism, there are numerous groups and foundations committed to raising awareness of and fighting for those affected by Brittle Bone Disease. These groups work together with medical experts, researchers, and lawmakers to create educational materials, carry out research, and advocate for legislative reforms that enhance the quality of life for people with brittle bone disease. These groups offer a crucial forum for people with Brittle Bone Disease to get together, share their experiences, and advocate for each other's rights.

The community is changing for the better thanks to the collaborative efforts of people with Brittle Bone Disease, medical professionals, researchers, and advocacy groups. They are enhancing the support systems accessible to persons with Brittle Bone Disease and enhancing their access to specialised care by sharing their stories, coordinating awareness campaigns, and fighting for policy reforms.

This subchapter has demonstrated the remarkable initiatives of people with brittle bone disease who are actively involved in raising awareness and advocating for change. These people are significantly enhancing the lives of persons who have Brittle Bone Disease through personal blogs, social media activity, organised support groups, and international campaigns. By telling their stories, spreading awareness, and fighting for legislative reforms, they are dispelling myths and enabling people with the illness to live happy, supportive lives. Their commitment and tenacity serve as an example to everyone, showing the value of collaboration, education, and advocacy in securing comprehensive healthcare for persons with Brittle Bone Disease.

Lessons Learned and Words of Wisdom

I have had the honour of working directly with people who have Brittle Bone Disease, commonly known as Osteogenesis Imperfecta, as a medical doctor and health and wellness coach. Each person's experiences and resiliency in the face of this difficult disease have taught me priceless lessons. I want to share some of these insights and advice in this chapter in the hopes that they will serve as motivation and direction for those going through comparable experiences.

Lesson 1: Embrace Your Unique Journey

Each person is affected differently by the complex disorder known as brittle bone disease. It is crucial to keep in mind that your path is distinct from the time of diagnosis. No two people will ever have the exact same experience, symptoms, or difficulties. You can handle the ups and downs with grace and resiliency by acknowledging this individuality and the possibility that your experience will be different from others.

Sarah, one of my patients, gave her opinion on the matter. She stated: "I was shocked and terrified when I first discovered what my illness was. But as time went on, I understood that my journey was unique. It was up to me to seize the opportunity and enjoy it. Instead of focusing on what I couldn't accomplish, I began to concentrate on what I could do and stopped making comparisons to other people."

Lesson 2: Find Your Support System

Brittle bone disease can be physically and psychologically difficult to live with. Forging a solid support network is essential to overcoming these obstacles. This support network could consist of close relatives, close friends, doctors, therapists, and other people who also have brittle bone disease.

Finding the appropriate support network was stressed by Jason, a patient I had the pleasure of working with. He stated: "Throughout my struggle, my family and friends have been my pillars of support. But I also got a lot of strength from interacting with people who related to my experience. Participating in support groups, going to conferences, and interacting with the internet community made me feel less alone and gave me essential encouragement and guidance."

Lesson 3: Educate Yourself and Advocate for Your Needs

When it comes to treating a challenging ailment like Brittle Bone Disease, knowledge truly is power. You can strengthen your ability to advocate for your needs by educating yourself on the most recent developments in therapies, treatments, and assistive technology.

A patient named Lindsay, who has battled brittle bone disease for more than 20 years, gave her perspective on the value of education. She stated: "I was determined to get knowledgeable about my situation. I was able to investigate many treatment options, have informed conversations with my doctors, and make decisions that were consistent with my goals and values because I had done my own research. Ask questions and get second viewpoints without hesitation. Your strongest ally is you."

Lesson 4: Focus on What You Can Control

Limitations and difficulties are frequently part of living with brittle bone disease. It is simple to become fixated on your limitations and lose sight of what you are capable of. To embrace your trip, it might make all the difference to change your viewpoint and focus on the things you can control.

Jessica, a patient who has figured out how to modify her way of life to fit her illness, gave some guidance. She stated: "I put more emphasis on my abilities and skills than on my shortcomings. I have looked into adaptive sports and discovered satisfaction in pursuits that I can engage in without risk. I have been able to live a full and busy life despite my illness by changing the way I think."

Lesson 5: Practice Self-Care and Prioritize Your Well-being

Maintaining both physical and mental well-being is crucial for those with brittle bone disease. To manage the difficulties and keep your general health, it is crucial to prioritise your well-being and engage in self-care.

A patient named Claire who adheres to holistic wellness methods underlined the value of self-care. She stated: "The need of looking after myself has become non-negotiable. This involves taking care of my body by eating wholesome foods, exercising frequently, and getting enough rest. But it also entails feeding my mind and spirit by meditating, going to therapy, and doing things I enjoy. Self-care is not selfish; it is essential to living a happy life."

Lesson 6: Embrace the Power of Resilience

Brittle Bone Disease demands a great deal of perseverance to live with. It's essential to have the capacity to overcome challenges, find courage when things get tough, and keep going forward.

Josh, a patient who has undergone numerous operations and fractures, offered his storey of resiliency. He stated: "The obstacles and difficulties I've encountered have put me to the test in ways I never anticipated. But they have also made me realise how incredibly strong I am. I keep my resilience in mind each time I face a challenge. It gives me the determination to press on and never give up."

Words of Wisdom:

In addition to these insightful lessons, people with Brittle Bone Disease also gave some advice for those dealing with comparable difficulties:

1 "Recognize that your illness does not determine who you are. You are much more than just your fragility." - Carly 2. "Celebrate your journey's milestones and minor successes. While to some they may appear unimportant, to you they serve as evidence of your fortitude and tenacity." - David 3. "Never hesitate to seek assistance. It requires courage to accept your limitations and help others." - Emma 4. "Associate yourself with inspiring and upbeat people who have faith in your abilities and support you." - Ryan 5. "Be kind to your body and yourself. Resting and taking care of yourself is OK since healing takes

time." - Maya 6. "Despite the suffering and difficulties, find the beauty in the journey. We discover our greatest strength during the difficult times in life, which are a sequence of ups and downs." - Ethan

In conclusion, having brittle bone disease creates certain difficulties, but it also brings chances for development, resiliency, and self-discovery. Brittle Bone Disease sufferers can travel their journey with grace and courage by accepting the lessons discovered and the advice offered by those who have gone before them. Keep in mind that you are not alone and that, despite its difficulties, your journey is ripe with opportunities for development and fulfilment.

Chapter 9: Supporting Friends and Family

Educating Yourself About Brittle Bone Disease

I have personally witnessed the effects that knowledge can have on patients and their families as a medical doctor and health and wellness coach. Understanding the illness is essential for appropriate therapy and support of osteogenesis imperfecta (OI), often known as brittle bone disease. You can assist your loved ones in navigating the difficulties of dealing with this uncommon genetic illness by arming yourself with knowledge.

It is critical to obtain reliable information about Brittle Bone Disease before you begin your educational path. Reputable medical websites and groups that focus on uncommon diseases are among the best places to start. You can find reliable and current information regarding the ailment on these sites, including details on its causes, types, symptoms, diagnosis, and available treatments. They might also provide you with educational materials and resources for support groups so you can learn more about the illness.

In addition to using online resources, speaking with medical experts who treat Brittle Bone Disease can be beneficial. These professionals, including paediatricians, geneticists, and orthopaedic surgeons, have specialised training and experience in treating this problem. They can answer any questions you may have and give you comprehensive information about the illness. Building a solid rapport with these experts might give you greater confidence to support your loved ones and fight for their medical requirements.

Patients and their families may struggle to cope with a chronic illness like brittle bone disease. Therefore, it's crucial to educate yourself about the condition's medical implications as well as its psychosocial and emotional effects. You can better support and empathise with your loved ones if you are aware of the emotional difficulties they are experiencing.

I will go in-depth on these facets of brittle bone disease in this section and provide management techniques for the condition's psychological and emotional effects. I'll talk about how open dialogue, attentive listening, and empathy help to foster emotional well-being. In addition, I'll talk about coping mechanisms that can be useful for patients and their families as they deal with the ups and downs of having brittle bone disease.

Investigating complementary and alternative therapies that could help with the management of Brittle Bone Disease symptoms can also be beneficial. These therapies can give your loved ones extra support, while they should always be used in addition to standard medical care. Techniques including physiotherapy, occupational therapy, and hydrotherapy may enhance mobility, muscle strength, and quality of life in general. I'll talk about various therapies, their possible advantages, and how to include them in an all-encompassing therapy strategy.

It is essential to involve your loved ones in their own care and decision-making processes in order to better support them. Encourage them to express their concerns and desires and actively engage in their treatment plan. You can help them feel more in charge and enhance their general well-being by giving them the tools they need to actively manage their health.

It can be useful to educate others in your community as well as yourself on Brittle Bone Disease. Increasing knowledge and understanding of the condition can help people with Brittle Bone Disease feel less stigmatised, receive more assistance, and live in a more welcoming environment. I'll offer advice and tips on how to effectively support your loved ones and raise awareness of the condition.

You will have a thorough grasp of Brittle Bone Disease at the end of this subchapter, as well as the skills required to be an understanding and helpful caregiver. You will have access to helpful tools, trustworthy data, and techniques for comprehending and managing the illness. Your loved ones will gain from this information, and it will also help you make wise choices and give your family the finest care possible.

Always keep in mind that learning is a journey, and this chapter will give you a solid understanding of brittle bone disease. Armed with information, empathy, and support, everyone of us can help to demystify this condition and improve the lives of individuals who are afflicted by it.

Communication and Active Listening

As a physician and health and wellness coach, I have firsthand experience with the difficulties that people with brittle bone disease have on a daily basis. In addition to the physical restrictions imposed by their illness, they also have to overcome several social and mental obstacles. Here, the assistance of friends and family is essential.

According to my observations, good communication is essential to creating a welcoming and understanding environment for people who have Brittle Bone Disease. We may provide them the emotional support they require while still fostering their independence and self-worth by being careful with our words and deeds.

Open discourse is one of the most crucial components of effective communication. It is crucial to establish a secure environment where people with Brittle Bone Disease can communicate their ideas, worries, and concerns without fear of rejection or criticism. We must listen attentively to this. We frequently have a tendency to offer our own suggestions or thoughts without really hearing what others have to say. We may make sure that their words are heard and their feelings are acknowledged by engaging in active listening.

Being in the moment and paying close attention to the speaker are both components of active listening. It entails putting down outside distractions like phones or other gadgets in order to fully concentrate on the person in front of us. We can communicate to someone that we are totally involved in the conversation by maintaining eye contact and utilising appropriate body language, such as nodding or leaning in.

Another crucial element of good communication is empathy. It requires putting ourselves in the patient's shoes and attempting to see things from their point of view. Even if we are unable to fully understand their experiences, we must acknowledge and respect their feelings. By demonstrating empathy, we foster an atmosphere of compassion and understanding.

It is crucial to speak positively and refrain from making assumptions or judgments while interacting with people who have Brittle Bone Disease. It is important to recognise each person's individuality because every person's experience with the illness is different. We can modify our sentences to be more empowering and encouraging rather than saying, "You can't do that," by asking, "Have you considered this alternative?" or "Let's find a method for you to accomplish that goal."

Education is a crucial component of good communication. Friends and family members of people with Brittle Bone Disease should become knowledgeable about the ailment, its signs and symptoms, and the difficulties it can present. They will be more equipped to offer support thanks to this expertise, which will also improve communication. We can better customise our communication to the requirements of people with Brittle Bone Disease if we are aware of the physical restrictions and potential consequences they experience.

Effective communication also heavily relies on non-verbal cues in addition to verbal communication. People who have brittle bone disease frequently have restricted mobility or may utilise aids like wheelchairs or crutches. It's crucial to pay attention to our body language and make sure that our gestures and expressions are respectful and inclusive. Simple but thoughtful actions can go a long way, such as making room for their mobility aids, using the proper seating arrangements, and being patient and understanding when they need more time.

Effective communication methods are necessary, but it's also crucial to take into account how Brittle Bone Disease affects people's relationships with their loved ones emotionally. Being sympathetic and understanding is necessary, but it's also critical to give them the coping mechanisms and assistance they require to get through the emotional difficulties.

Friends and family of people with Brittle Bone Disease may find it helpful to join support groups, both offline and online. These organisations offer a forum for exchanging experiences, getting suggestions, and receiving emotional support from people in related circumstances. It can be immensely powerful and comforting to make a connection with those who have experienced the particular difficulties of living with brittle bone disease.

It's important to look after our own mental and emotional health as friends and family members. Supporting people with Brittle Bone Disease can occasionally be emotionally taxing. Finding appropriate outlets for our own emotions, scheduling time for self-care, and going to therapy or counselling are all crucial aspects in preserving our own mental wellbeing. We can better assist our loved ones on their journey if we do this.

In summary, encouraging a friendly and understanding environment for people with Brittle Bone Disease requires excellent communication and active listening. We may foster an environment that fosters their independence, self-esteem, and general well-being by engaging in active listening, demonstrating empathy, using positive language, learning about the condition, being aware of nonverbal clues, and offering emotional support. Together, let's use good communication and active listening to empower and inspire those who have brittle bone disease.

Providing Emotional Support

This chapter will examine the many methods for offering emotional support to family members who have brittle bone disease. It can be difficult to live with this condition, both physically and emotionally, therefore your support will be essential to their overall wellbeing. We'll discuss a range of subjects, including empathising with others, being validated, and fostering a welcoming workplace.

1. Validation: Recognizing and Acknowledging Feelings

Validation is one of the most crucial components of offering emotional support. Frustration, sadness, and worry are just a few of the various feelings that people with brittle bone disease may feel. In order to reassure them that their feelings are legitimate and reasonable, it is crucial to acknowledge and validate them.

You can start by actively and nonjudgmentally listening as a caregiver or loved one. Allow them to openly express their feelings without being interrupted or discounted. Avoid sayings that could minimise their sentiments, such as "You shouldn't feel that way" or "Don't be so depressed." Rather, attempt to mirror back to them their feelings by saying something like, "It sounds like you're feeling particularly disappointed with the limits imposed by the sickness.."

2. Empathy: Understanding Their Perspective

Having empathy is a crucial characteristic while offering emotional support. You must strive to understand the world from your loved one's point of view in order to fully comprehend what they are going through. Empathy enables you to offer consolation and assistance in light of their particular struggles and experiences.

It's critical to keep in mind that you cannot fully comprehend the suffering and difficulties associated with having brittle bone disease when engaging in empathy. Instead, make an effort to pay attention and pick up new information while demonstrating sincere care in their welfare. Don't minimise their experiences or compare them to others because doing so could invalidate their emotions. Instead, sincerely inquire about how they are feeling and extend an unbiased ear.

3. Creating a Safe and Inclusive Environment

For people with Brittle Bone Disease to experience emotional well-being, it is essential to provide a secure and welcoming atmosphere. Making their physical and social environments hospitable and accessible is necessary to achieve this. Here are some crucial things to remember:

a. Physical Safety: It is crucial to make sure that the physical setting is secure and welcoming. Eliminate any dangers or barriers that could cause harm. To accommodate their particular needs, modify the living areas by adding grab bars or ramps, for example. You can lessen the ongoing anxiety about future accidents by taking these proactive measures.

b. Social Inclusion: Due to the physical restrictions of their condition, people with brittle bone disease may frequently feel alone. It is crucial to establish social settings where kids can experience inclusion and value. Encourage loved ones and friends to get together frequently in welcoming environments by making sure that events and gathering places are open to everyone. Their emotional health can be dramatically impacted by creating a sense of acceptance and belonging.

c. Education and Awareness: Encourage a culture of knowledge and awareness about brittle bone disease in your immediate social circle and the larger society. This can foster better comprehension and support while helping to eliminate myths. Encourage the person you care about to speak up for their needs and share their experiences. You can help create a society that is more compassionate and inclusive by spreading awareness.

4. Nurturing Emotional Resilience

It's important to build emotional resilience because having brittle bone disease can be emotionally taxing. Emotional resilience is the capacity to deal with adversity, recover from failures, and keep a positive attitude in the face of difficulties. Here are some methods for fostering emotional toughness:

a. Mindfulness and Relaxation Techniques: To increase emotional well-being, incorporate mindfulness and relaxation practises into regular activities. Encourage your loved one to practise practises like writing, deep breathing, or meditation. These methods can assist individuals in handling stress, lowering anxiety, and keeping a more impartial viewpoint.

b. Self-Care and Self-Compassion: Help your loved one make self-care a priority. This includes pursuits that make them happy, comfortable, and fulfilled. Encourage them to take up hobbies, make friends who will support them, and learn self-compassion. Remind them that prioritising their emotional health and taking breaks are both acceptable.

c. Building a Support Network: Encourage your loved one to look for help from people who understand their situation. This could entail connecting with people who have the same conditions or joining support groups or online forums. Being empowered by others' stories and guidance can make them feel less alone in their path..

d. Seeking Professional Help: It may be helpful to seek professional assistance if a loved one is having emotional difficulties. Encourage them to get in touch with a therapist or counsellor who focuses on disabilities or chronic illnesses. Professional assistance can offer more direction and resources to help people through the emotional difficulties brought on by Brittle Bone Disease.

Conclusion: A Journey of Emotional Support

It takes time and effort to support someone who has brittle bone disease emotionally. It necessitates compassion, comprehension, and a dedication to fostering a welcoming workplace. Keep in mind that each person's experience with the condition is distinct, and that you can help them deal by showing your support and empathy.

Your loved one can acquire the skills to control their emotions and thrive in spite of the difficulties they encounter by fostering emotional resilience and promoting self-care. Communicate with them honestly and openly, and urge them to contact a professional if necessary.

By working together, we can improve the emotional health of people with brittle bone disease..

Practical Assistance and Accommodations

Adapting the Environment:

Making changes to the environment to ensure safety and accessibility is one of the first stages in providing practical support. Brittle bone disease patients are extremely prone to fractures, so it's important that their surroundings are risk-free. This can entail tripping hazards like loose carpets, furniture with sharp edges, and other things like that being removed or secured. It can be helpful to provide support and stability by installing grab bars and handrails in important locations like bathrooms and stairways.

Additionally, it could be required to alter the home's design to meet the special requirements of those who have Brittle Bone Disease. This can entail adding ramps for simpler access to various parts of the property, enlarging entrances to allow wheelchairs or walkers, and altering the height of counters and bookcases to make them more accessible.

Assisting with Daily Activities:

Even the most routine everyday tasks can be difficult for someone with brittle bone disease. It is our duty as healthcare providers to provide reasonable adjustments and hands-on support to make it easier for people with Brittle Bone Disease to go about their everyday lives.

Personal care activities including bathing, clothing, and grooming are one area where assistance is frequently required. Give patients adaptable tools like long-handled brushes or sponges to help them reach hard-to-reach places. To improve stability and safety when bathing, grab bars and handheld showerheads can be installed in the bathroom.

The incidence of fractures can also be significantly decreased by providing instruction on good body mechanics and methods for transferring to and from chairs, beds, and other surfaces. This could entail making arrangements for the installation of chair lifts or stair lifts to help with mobility or instructing patients on how to use assistive devices like transfer boards or slide sheets.

Promoting Independence:

The promotion of independence for those with Brittle Bone Disease is just as vital as providing practical help. This can significantly enhance their sense of self-worth and general well-being.

Encouraging people with Brittle Bone Disease to engage in physical activities that are suitable for their condition is one strategy to enhance independence. This may entail collaborating closely with occupational therapists and physical therapists to create personalised training regimens that promote bone density, strengthen muscles, and improve range of motion. People with Brittle Bone Disease can enhance their general physical health and lower their risk of fractures by participating in regular physical activity.

Additionally, offering educational materials and support systems can aid those who have brittle bone disease in better understanding their condition and discovering practical coping mechanisms. This can entail linking them with online communities or support groups where they can share their stories and get advice from those going through comparable struggles. Giving advice on stress reduction methods, mindfulness exercises, and relaxation techniques can also assist people with Brittle Bone Disease maintain their emotional health and manage the pressures of having a chronic illness.

Conclusion:

I've given advice on how to give support and accommodations in the real world to people with brittle bone disease in this chapter. We can considerably enhance the quality of life for persons with this condition by making the environment more accommodating, providing assistance with everyday tasks, and encouraging independence. I am convinced that individuals with brittle bone disease are capable of overcoming the restrictions placed on them by their illness and leading happy, self-sufficient lives with the help of medical specialists. Let's work together to dispel myths about brittle bone disease and provide people the tools they need to live life to the fullest.

Fostering Inclusivity and Advocacy

I sincerely think that promoting inclusivity is not only the healthcare system's job but also a group effort on the part of society as a whole. I am a doctor and a health and wellness coach. It is essential to foster an atmosphere where people who have Brittle Bone Disease feel supported, comprehended, and included. I'll walk you through some doable actions you can do to advance activism and inclusivity in this section.

Educating Yourself

Educating oneself is the first and most important step in promoting inclusivity and acting as an advocate for people with Brittle Bone Disease. Become as knowledgeable as you can about the illness, its causes, symptoms, and effects on the person's life. Recognize the difficulties they confront and any particular requirements they may have. You will be better able to combat misunderstandings, stereotypes, and stigmas connected with Brittle Bone Disease if you have a thorough grasp of the condition.

Promoting Awareness

It's essential to spread knowledge about brittle bone disease in order to promote inclusivity and build a welcoming neighbourhood. To disseminate knowledge about the disease, use a variety of outlets, including social media, neighbourhood activities, and educational seminars. To plan awareness campaigns and presentations, work with the nearby colleges, hospitals, and schools. By educating people about the condition, you can help dispel misconceptions and promote compassion and understanding.

Challenging Stigma

Stigma frequently results from ignorance or incorrect information. As advocates, it is our responsibility to dispel these stereotypes and advance an inclusive society. Start by addressing prevalent myths regarding brittle bone disease and debunking them with factual information. Share your own experiences and those of people with the disease who have achieved achievement in a variety of spheres of life. Draw attention to their fortitude and accomplishments to illustrate that brittle bone disease does not define them.

Creating a Supportive Community

To thrive, people with Brittle Bone Disease must create a supportive community. Encourage the establishment of support groups so that people with the condition can interact, exchange stories, and find comfort in a secure setting. These groups can offer beneficial emotional support and useful guidance on dealing with day-to-day difficulties. Promote neighbourhood gatherings and activities for people with brittle bone disease and their loved ones. We can build a community that embraces diversity by encouraging a sense of support and belonging.

Encouraging Accessibility

Fostering inclusivity depends on accessibility. Advocate for improving accessibility for people with mobility issues brought on by Brittle Bone Disease in public areas, on public transportation, and at work. Advocate for laws and regulations that mandate that all buildings be accessible to those using wheelchairs, with ramps and elevators always available. Encourage nearby companies to offer facilities for people with disabilities, such as wide entrances, accessible restrooms, and special parking spots. We can guarantee equitable chances for people with brittle bone disease by advocating for accessibility.

Providing Resources and Support

As advocates, it is our responsibility to give people with Brittle Bone Disease the tools and encouragement they need to live happy, full lives. This can entail putting patients in touch with medical experts familiar with the illness, pain-management specialists, and assistive technology that improves mobility and independence. assist people in navigating the healthcare system, comprehending insurance coverage, and obtaining financial aid. Bridging the gap between those in need and resources will enable those with brittle bone disease to thrive.

Engaging in Policy Advocacy

Policy advocacy is crucial if one hopes to effect long-lasting change. Work together with regional and national groups to promote laws that defend the rights and interests of people with disabilities, particularly those who suffer from Brittle Bone Disease. Encourage lawmakers to pass legislation that supports equity, accessibility, and inclusiveness in healthcare, employment, and education. Attend public forums, write letters to legislators, and speak up to support community issues. We can bring about systemic improvements that benefit all people with Brittle Bone Disease by actively engaging in policy advocacy.

Conclusion:

In order to promote inclusivity and work as an advocate for people with Brittle Bone Disease, one must be kind and proactive. We may have a big impact on the lives of persons afflicted by this condition by educating ourselves, raising awareness, combating stigma, building a supportive community, increasing accessibility, offering resources and assistance, and participating in legislative advocacy. Let's work together to create a world that embraces diversity and fights for everyone's rights and wellbeing, regardless of their health.

Chapter 10: Research and Advances in Brittle Bone Disease

Current Research Studies and Clinical Trials

Understanding the underlying genetic abnormalities that cause Brittle Bone Disease is one of the main areas of research in this field. Genes that are important for bone growth and remodelling have been found in several investigations. Understanding these genetic markers can aid in early disease diagnosis and offer more specialised therapy options.

For instance, a recent study by a group of scientists from Newcastle University's Institute of Genetic Medicine focused on finding unusual genetic abnormalities in people with Brittle Bone Disease. They were able to identify particular mutations that contribute to the disease by analysing the full exome, which comprises all of the coding areas of genes in our DNA. This discovery could pave the way for genetic counselling and testing, giving Brittle Bone Disease sufferers the information they need to make decisions about their health and the chance of passing the disease on to future generations.

Investigating the possible application of stem cell therapy for the treatment of brittle bone disease is another area of active research. The extraordinary capacity of stem cells to develop into several cell types, including bone cells. Researchers are now examining whether these cells can be used to repair damaged bone structures and increase bone strength in people with brittle bone disease as a result of this.

The University of Edinburgh is currently conducting a ground-breaking clinical trial to test the effectiveness of employing bone marrow-derived stem cells to treat brittle bone disease. Participants in this study receive direct injections of their own stem cells into the damaged bone locations. The goal is to increase bone regeneration and decrease fracture incidence. Participants in the study showed better bone density and a decline in fracture incidence, which are promising preliminary results.

Many investigations are focused on creating pharmacological therapies for Brittle Bone Disease in addition to genetic research and stem cell therapy. Currently, the usage of bisphosphonates, a class of medications that aid in bone strength, is crucial for the management of the disease. Long-term usage of these drugs, however, may have negative effects, including gastrointestinal issues and a higher risk of atypical fractures. As a result, scientists are looking at other therapy modalities that might provide comparable advantages but with fewer adverse effects.

One such study is looking into the use of romosozumab, a monoclonal antibody that targets a protein involved in controlling bone remodelling. Romosozumab can aid in boosting bone production and lowering bone resorption by inhibiting this protein. Phase 3 clinical trials have thus far produced promising results, with participants reporting higher bone densities and a lower incidence of fractures.

Additionally, scientists are looking into the possibility of using gene therapy to cure brittle bone disease. To fix the underlying genetic mutation, gene therapy entails inserting healthy copies of the defective gene into cells. This strategy has enormous potential for the treatment of hereditary diseases like Brittle Bone Disease, including management and perhaps even cure.

Researchers at the Max Planck Institute for Molecular Biomedicine in Germany recently examined the potential of gene therapy to treat mice with brittle bone disease. After successfully introducing a corrected gene into the cells in charge of bone growth, the strength and durability of bones significantly increased. Even though this research is still in its early phases, it offers promising opportunities for the treatment of Brittle Bone Disease in people in the future.

Patients with Brittle Bone Disease and their families have the chance to advance medical science and maybe gain access to the most cutting-edge treatments by taking part in clinical studies. It is crucial to speak with your doctor and look into the local clinical trials that are offered. To protect the participants' safety and welfare, these experiments are strictly regulated.

In conclusion, the management of Brittle Bone Disease has a great deal of potential to be changed by the present research studies and clinical trials. Scientists and researchers are always working to increase our understanding of the condition and create more efficient treatment choices, including anything from genetic studies and stem cell therapy to pharmaceutical interventions and gene therapy. People with Brittle Bone Disease can take control of their health and investigate the possibility of taking part in clinical trials by learning more about the current research and potential future developments. It is our duty as medical professionals to stay current on these ground-breaking advancements and provide the best treatment to our patients. Together, we can dispel the mystery surrounding brittle bone disease and open the door to a better future for individuals who are afflicted with it.

Genetic Discoveries and Therapeutic Targets

Understanding the genetic causes of Brittle Bone Disease has advanced significantly over time. We now understand that COL1A1 and COL1A2 gene mutations are the primary causes of the disease. The alpha chains of type I collagen, a protein essential for the composition and durability of bones, are encoded by these genes. Type I collagen is produced, assembled, or stabilised by these genes, therefore mutations in these genes can affect these processes, resulting in weaker and brittle bones.

Through thorough investigation, researchers have discovered more than 200 distinct mutations in the COL1A1 and COL1A2 genes, each of which contributes to the onset of Brittle Bone Disease. While some mutations result in a less drastic decrease in collagen formation, others cause the complete absence of type I collagen. The clinical signs of the condition, which can range in severity from mild to severe, are frequently determined by the kind and severity of the mutation.

The discovery of possible treatment targets is one of the most intriguing advancements in the study of brittle bone disease. Understanding the precise processes by which these genetic abnormalities reduce collagen formation has led researchers to consider novel therapeutic approaches to enhance bone health.

Use of bisphosphonates, a class of medications that prevents bone resorption and raises bone density, is one possible therapeutic strategy. According to studies, bisphosphonates can lower fracture rates and increase bone mineral density in people with brittle bone disease. It is crucial to remember that bisphosphonates may have side effects and may be less effective in people whose collagen production is weak or severe.

The modification of genes involved in the manufacture of collagen is another possible therapeutic target. Recent developments in gene therapy have made it possible to improve collagen production or correct genetic abnormalities in people with brittle bone disease. For instance, scientists have successfully corrected particular mutations in cells taken from patients with the condition using gene editing methods like CRISPR-Cas9. Although this strategy is still in its infancy, it has a lot of potential for future therapeutic choices.

Furthermore, research has demonstrated that specific growth factors, including bone morphogenetic proteins (BMPs) and transforming growth factor-beta (TGF-), are essential for the production and regeneration of bone. Researchers seek to create treatments that can stimulate bone development and enhance bone strength in people with brittle bone disease by focusing on these growth factors. Although preliminary findings from animal studies have showed encouraging results, more investigation is required to determine the safety and effectiveness of such therapies.

The necessity of holistic treatment for people with Brittle Bone Disease must be emphasised in addition to these genetic discoveries and pharmacological targets. Healthcare practitioners advise patients on lifestyle changes, self-care methods, and coping mechanisms in addition to focusing on the biological elements of the disease.

For instance, individualised physical therapy and exercise programmes can aid in enhancing muscle strength, balance, and coordination, which lowers the chance of fractures. Interventions in occupational therapy can help people adjust to their physical limits and create plans for performing daily activities safely. The emotional and psychological effects of having a chronic illness like Brittle Bone Disease must also be managed, which calls for therapy and psychological care.

In conclusion, there has been substantial advancement in the field of brittle bone disease research in terms of comprehending the genetic underpinnings of the condition and discovering prospective therapeutic targets. While improvements in gene therapy and the investigation of growth factor modification give hope for future treatments, the finding of mutations in the COL1A1 and COL1A2 genes has provided insight into the underlying mechanisms causing the disease.

However, it is crucial to approach the treatment of brittle bone disease holistically, taking into account lifestyle changes, self-care strategies, and psychological support in addition to genetic therapies. Combining these strategies will enable people with brittle bone disease to live fulfilling lives while coping with the problems the condition presents.

Healthcare practitioners must keep current and work with researchers, geneticists, and other specialists to provide the best care for people with Brittle Bone Disease as the field develops and new discoveries are made. Together, we can remove the mystery surrounding this ailment and open the door to a better future for all who are impacted.

Regenerative Medicine and Bone Repair

Chapter 7: Regenerative Medicine and Bone Repair

Both regenerative medicine and methods for repairing broken bones have made substantial strides in recent years. For those who have Osteogenesis Imperfecta, generally known as Brittle Bone Disease, these discoveries hold enormous potential. It is my responsibility as a medical professional and health and wellness coach to make the public aware of the most recent advancements in this field, as well as the guiding principles that underlie these methods and their potential to enhance bone health.

Bone is an extraordinary tissue with some degree of self-healing abilities. The body's capacity to repair and regenerate bone is jeopardised in the case of brittle bone disease. Due to this inherited condition, the bones are brittle and easily break with even the smallest pressure or impact. Living with this illness can result in a never-ending cycle of pain, loneliness, and constrained mobility.

Fortunately, people with Brittle Bone Disease now have new hope thanks to regenerative medicine. A promising treatment approach has developed in particular for stem cell therapy. Undifferentiated cells called stem cells have the remarkable capacity to differentiate into many distinct cell types, including bone cells. Researchers have been able to promote bone tissue growth and regeneration by utilising the power of stem cells.

Mesenchymal stem cells (MSCs) are injected into the patient's body as one method of stem cell treatment. MSCs come from many different places, including bone marrow, adipose tissue, and umbilical cord blood. These cells have exceptional regeneration powers and have the capacity to develop into multiple cell types, including osteoblasts, which build bones.

These MSCs migrate to the location of bone damage or injury after being injected into the patient. Here, they start the process of differentiation, developing into osteoblasts and assisting in bone tissue repair. This regenerative strategy offers a way to not only fix broken bones but also strengthen the entire skeletal framework, which has huge potential for those with Brittle Bone Disease.

Growth factors and scaffolds are used in regenerative medicine as yet another cutting-edge method to speed up bone healing. Growth factors are organic proteins that control cellular differentiation and growth. Researchers have discovered a way to enhance the body's generation of bone cells and quicken the mending process by injecting particular growth factors into the body.

Scaffolds are essential in bone repair together with growth factors. The scaffolding provided by scaffold materials serves to facilitate the development of new bone tissue. These scaffolds can be created using a number of materials, including collagen, ceramics, and synthetic polymers. Scaffolds improve the efficiency of regenerative therapies by giving bone cells a structure to regenerate in.

Additionally, new gene therapy research opens up fresh options for the treatment of brittle bone disease. Gene therapy involves introducing healthy genes directly into the patient's cells or using a vector, such a virus, to do so. This strategy seeks to fix the underlying genetic alterations that gave rise to the disease.

Scientists hope to improve bone strength by focusing on the specific genes linked to brittle bone disease and restoring the natural function of bone cells. Although gene therapy is still in its infancy, it has great promise for the future and might offer a long-term cure for this crippling condition.

While these developments in bone repair and regenerative medicine give hope to people with brittle bone disease, it's crucial to remember that more studies and clinical trials are required to confirm their safety and efficacy. As a doctor, I firmly believe in the practise of evidence-based medicine and advise patients to approach these novel treatments with caution and under the direction of professionals.

In conclusion, people with brittle bone disease have a lot of hope for the future thanks to advances in regenerative medicine and bone repair procedures. Gene therapy, scaffolds, growth factors, and stem cell therapy are just a few of the cutting-edge techniques being investigated in this area. These developments have the potential to improve the entire skeletal system in addition to healing broken bones. However, it is crucial to use caution while using these medicines and to hold off until additional studies and clinical trials can confirm their efficacy. We may anticipate better bone health and a better future for people with brittle bone disease because to ongoing developments in regenerative medicine.

Assistive Technologies and Accessibility Innovations

When it comes to helping people with Brittle Bone Disease move around safely, mobility aids are essential. To better serve these people's unique demands, traditional mobility aids like wheelchairs and walkers have received substantial improvements. There are now lightweight wheelchairs designed specifically for those with Brittle Bone Disease. These wheelchairs are made to be cosy, sturdy, and offer the best support possible to reduce the danger of fractures. These wheelchairs may also be folded up and transported with ease, allowing people to continue living active lives.

Additionally, improvements in adaptive technology have fundamentally changed how people with Brittle Bone Disease perform their daily duties. One of these advancements was the creation of reachers and grabbers, which allow people to pick up items from the floor or high shelves without putting an undue amount of stress on their bones. These gadgets are made to be light and comfortable to hold, giving users more independence when going about their daily lives. To address the weak grip strength frequently associated with Brittle Bone Disease, adaptive eating utensils with wider handles and altered shapes have also been created. These tools guarantee that people may eat comfortably and safely on their own, fostering a sense of independence and dignity.

Another area that has made considerable strides recently is inclusive design. The goal of inclusive design is to provide goods and places that are usable by individuals with a variety of skills and limitations. Architects and designers can make sure that structures, public areas, and transportation systems are accessible to people with Brittle Bone Disease by using universal design principles. For those with limited mobility, putting handrails in public areas, building ramps with gentle slopes in place of steps, and designing doors that are simple to open and close can all significantly improve accessibility.

The lives of people with Brittle Bone Disease have been significantly improved by technology. Electric scooters and wheelchairs are examples of powered mobility equipment that have progressed and now offer better control and manoeuvrability. Individuals can more easily explore a variety of terrains and situations thanks to these technologies, which increases their opportunities for social interaction and involvement in a range of activities.

Additionally, technologically advanced assistive gadgets have been created to give people more freedom and convenience in their daily lives, such as voice-activated home automation systems. Those with limited mobility due to Brittle Bone Disease can experience enhanced autonomy inside their homes by using voice commands to manage the lights, temperature, and other home appliances.

The quality of life for those with Brittle Bone Disease has been significantly improved as a result of advances in prosthetic technology. Specific prosthetic limbs made for people with weak bones provide the best support while maintaining comfort and functionality. Each person's unique anatomical requirements can be taken into account when creating custom prosthetics, giving them a more natural range of motion and lowering their risk of injury.

Additionally, 3D printing has grown to be a potent tool in the assistive technology industry. With the use of this technology, medical practitioners can now design individualised assistive and adaptive equipment that is specifically suited to the needs of people with brittle bone disease. In addition to offering improved support and stability to weak bones, 3D-printed braces and splints also guarantee a pleasant fit. People with Brittle Bone Disease now have a much higher quality of life thanks to the ability to design personalised solutions using 3D printing.

In conclusion, accessibility advances and the development of assistive technologies have fundamentally changed how people with Brittle Bone Disease go about their daily lives. Accessibility has been substantially improved thanks to mobility aids, adaptive technology, and inclusive design, allowing people with this disability to participate in society on an equal basis. People now have more independence and convenience because to technology, such as motorised mobility aids and voice-activated home automation systems. Furthermore, improvements in prosthetics and 3D printing have led to the creation of personalised solutions that better meet the particular requirements of people with Brittle Bone Disease. Future developments in assistive technologies for people with Brittle Bone Disease hold even more promise as medical professionals and academics continue to collaborate and create, giving them the chance to lead satisfying and independent lives.

Future Directions and Hope

I've always had a great belief in the potential of innovation and teamwork in the medical industry. Numerous improvements have been achieved in the knowledge, identification, and management of Brittle Bone Disease over time. These developments have created new opportunities for better disease management and given patients hope for a better future.

The creation of innovative therapeutics for Brittle Bone Disease is one area of ongoing research that shows considerable potential. Understanding the underlying genetic underpinnings of the disease has advanced significantly in recent years. This has made it possible to investigate specialised treatments and interventions meant to target the particular genetic defects causing the weaker bone structure.

In preclinical research and preliminary clinical trials, cutting-edge procedures like gene therapy and stem cell transplantation have showed promise. These methods aim to restore normal bone strength and avoid fractures by trying to replace or correct the defective genes that cause brittle bone disease. Though they are still in the research and development stages, these cutting-edge therapies give patients with brittle bone disease hope that they may one day be able to lead more active and fracture-free lives.

The creation of efficient pharmaceutical therapies to improve bone strength in people with Brittle Bone Disease is another area of study emphasis. The main method of addressing the problem has been with traditional therapies such bisphosphonates and calcium supplements, however these are not always successful. Researchers are currently looking into new therapeutic targets that could provide better results, such as the creation of drugs that can encourage bone production and block bone resorption.

There is rising interest in the use of complementary and alternative therapies for people with Brittle Bone Disease beyond the sphere of conventional medicine. These therapeutic modalities, which include exercises like yoga, meditation, and acupuncture, can aid with pain management, flexibility enhancement, and general well-being. By include these methods in the regimen, doctors can provide patients more tools to deal with the mental and physical difficulties of having the disease.

Furthermore, it is critical to recognise the value of teamwork and interdisciplinary methods in the treatment of people with Brittle Bone Disease in the future. The problem is intricate and multidimensional, necessitating the knowledge of numerous medical specialists. A multidisciplinary strategy involving, among others, orthopaedic surgeons, endocrinologists, physiotherapists, geneticists, psychiatrists, and nutritionists is required to ensure thorough and holistic therapy.

Collaboration has the capacity to satisfy the many requirements of patients and provide a more comprehensive view of their entire health. This could entail developing customised programmes that address the particular difficulties faced by people with Brittle Bone Disease, as well as coordinating treatment regimens, sharing knowledge and expertise, and other strategies. Healthcare workers can pool their resources, share ideas, and give patients the greatest care by cooperating.

In addition, technology will continue to have a major impact on how Brittle Bone Disease is managed in the future. Modern imaging methods, such as whole-body MRI and high-resolution CT scans, enable earlier disease diagnosis and more precise disease progression monitoring. With the aid of these technologies, medical personnel can now detect fractures, analyse bone density, and evaluate the efficacy of various treatment options in real time.

For those with brittle bone disease, the rise of wearable technology, including smartwatches and activity trackers, offers intriguing new prospects. These tools can detect indications of bone health, track levels of physical activity, and give feedback on safe movement techniques. Utilizing technology allows individuals to take an active role in their own care, preventing fractures and maintaining overall bone health.

Along with improvements in medical research and technology, it's critical to give people with Brittle Bone Disease the support and knowledge they need to succeed in daily life. This can be accomplished by providing patients with focused educational programmes that teach them about bone health, fracture prevention methods, and self-care practises. Their general well-being and quality of life can be considerably improved by psychological assistance, counselling, and coping mechanisms.

The future is ultimately full with hope for those who have Brittle Bone Disease. We can imagine a time when the effects of the disease are reduced and people can live full and active lives thanks to continued research, teamwork, and an integrated approach to care. Even though there is still much to be done, the progress that has been accomplished thus far shows great potential and gives patients, their families, and healthcare professionals alike cause for optimism.

I am dedicated to being on the cutting edge of these developments and giving my patients the finest care possible in my capacity as a medical doctor and health and wellness coach. I work to provide a thorough and individualised approach to managing Brittle Bone Disease with the help of my team of professionals from various health and wellness sectors. We want to give each patient the tools they need to manage their path with hope and resiliency by attending to their physical, emotional, and psychological needs.

In conclusion, cutting-edge research, professional teamwork, technological developments, and a wholistic approach to care are the cornerstones of the future directions and hope for people with brittle bone disease. The progress accomplished thus far gives us hope, knowing that each step taken puts us closer to a future in which people with Brittle Bone Disease can live their lives to the fullest, even though the path ahead may still be littered with challenges.

Chapter 11: Building a Supportive Healthcare Team

Identifying the Right Healthcare Professionals

Selecting Specialists:

Choosing the appropriate specialists is the first step in locating the best medical personnel. Osteogenesis Imperfecta, another name for the rare genetic illness known as brittle bone disease, impairs the body's capacity to make collagen, leaving patients with brittle, easily fractured bones. Professionals with experience in several facets of Osteogenesis Imperfecta are needed to manage this disorder.

One of the most crucial specialists to take into account is an orthopaedic surgeon with knowledge of treating patients with Brittle Bone Disease. Orthopedic surgeons are skilled at identifying and treating musculoskeletal issues and can provide helpful advice on how to handle fractures and complications involving the bones. Choose a surgeon who has a proven track record and a wealth of experience treating patients with this uncommon illness.

A geneticist should also be a member of the medical staff. Doctors who specialise in diagnosing genetic abnormalities are known as geneticists, and they can provide genetic testing and counselling to people with Brittle Bone Disease. They can assist people comprehend the inheritance pattern and possible hazards for future generations, as well as offer insights into the condition's underlying aetiology.

Brittle Bone Disease can be effectively managed by a physiatrist with expertise in rehabilitation medicine. Through non-surgical interventions like physical therapy, occupational therapy, and pain management methods, physiatrists aim to enhance quality of life and general function. These experts can offer advice on physical activities, adaptable tools, and assistive gadgets that can help people with Brittle Bone Disease keep their independence and make the most of their physical capabilities.

A rheumatologist should also be consulted in addition to these specialists for people who have joint pain or other rheumatic symptoms linked to Brittle Bone Disease. Rheumatologists are medical professionals that focus on the identification and management of rheumatic diseases, particularly those that affect the bones, joints, and connective tissues. They can offer advice on drugs and other measures to treat these symptoms, and their experience can assist control the joint pain and inflammation that are frequently linked to Brittle Bone Disease.

Building a Multidisciplinary Team:

Building a multidisciplinary team that can collaborate to deliver complete treatment is just as vital as having the appropriate specialists. Brittle bone disease has an impact on a person's physical, emotional, and psychological well-being, among other elements of their life. Therefore, having personnel from several healthcare specialties who can handle these various demands is advantageous.

Consider adding a physical therapist or physiotherapist to the team in addition to the medical professionals already indicated. To help build stronger bones and increase mobility, they can offer specialised workouts and therapies that are adapted to the demands of the individual. By suggesting adaptable tools and techniques to get around the difficulties of Brittle Bone Disease, occupational therapists can also be extremely helpful in promoting independence and facilitating daily tasks.

The psychological and emotional effects of having a rare and difficult condition like Brittle Bone Disease can be managed with the help of psychologists or therapists that specialise in chronic sickness and disability. They can offer counselling, coping mechanisms, and methods for overcoming any potential emotional obstacles.

Accessing Comprehensive Care:

Accessibility to thorough care must be guaranteed once you have chosen the best medical specialists and assembled your multidisciplinary team. This calls for coordination between the various specialists, frequent follow-up appointments, and efficient teamwork.

The treatment obtained for controlling Brittle Bone Disease goes beyond just medical procedures. It involves a multifaceted strategy that considers factors in the physical, emotional, and psychological realms. Therefore, it is essential to create open lines of communication among the entire team to guarantee that the treatment given is coordinated and consistent.

It is important to schedule frequent follow-up appointments with each specialist to keep track of the patient's development, discuss any issues, and modify the treatment plan as appropriate. These checkups are essential for delaying and treating issues like joint pain and fractures, as well as for maintaining general health.

Individuals should have access to emergency medical treatment in addition to their routine appointments. With the possibility of fractures associated with brittle bone disease, it's critical to have a plan in place for rapid and proper care in case of emergency. This can entail locating musculoskeletal injury-capable hospitals or clinics in the area and building a rapport with medical professionals who are knowledgeable with the patient's condition.

Conclusion:

Finding the best healthcare providers for Brittle Bone Disease is essential for providing thorough care and achieving the best results in managing this uncommon ailment. People can create a multidisciplinary team that caters to their various needs by choosing doctors with training in orthopaedics, genetics, rehabilitation medicine, and rheumatology. These experts can offer comprehensive help and direction in managing the physical, emotional, and psychological components of Brittle Bone Disease, along with physiotherapists, occupational therapists, and psychologists. Additionally, it is crucial to create team member effectiveness and regular follow-up visits in order to provide accessibility to comprehensive care. By adopting these actions, those who have Brittle Bone Disease can get the finest care possible, enabling them to live happy lives despite the difficulties that come with their illness.

Effective Communication With Healthcare Providers

Definition and Context:

Having good communication is essential to receive high-quality medical care. It is crucial for patients to actively communicate with their healthcare professionals, raise any concerns they may have, and comprehend the decisions being made regarding their care. Effective communication is even more important when you have brittle bone disease because it enables you to speak up for your needs and get the best care possible.

I'll present helpful tips and strategies on how to interact with healthcare providers in this section. As a physician and health and wellness coach, I have seen that patients who actively participate in making healthcare decisions frequently enjoy better outcomes and feel more in control of their health journeys.

Asking Questions:

Knowing when and how to ask questions is one of the most important aspects of good communication with healthcare professionals. It is imperative to learn more and get any questions you might have answered regarding your illness, available treatments, or prognosis.

It is crucial to have a list of questions ready before speaking with your healthcare professional. By doing so, you can make sure you handle all the pertinent issues and any potential problems. You might think about posing the following inquiries:

What causes my brittle bones, and why? Is it inherited or brought on by other elements?

2. What medical alternatives are there for my particular condition?

3. What are the advantages and disadvantages of each therapy option?

4. Are there any complementary or alternative treatments that might be useful?

5. What alterations to my way of life may I do to better my bone health?

6. How will these procedures impact my general health and quality of life?

7. What can I anticipate for my condition's long-term prognosis and management?

You give yourself the power to make knowledgeable decisions about your healthcare by actively seeking information and posing pertinent questions. Keep in mind that when it comes to your wellbeing, no inquiry is too minor or unimportant.

Expressing Concerns:

It's important to voice your thoughts and concerns to your healthcare professionals in order to have effective communication. Sharing these feelings with your healthcare team will help them better understand your requirements and give you the assistance you need. It is common to feel frightened or overwhelmed after receiving a diagnosis of brittle bone disease.

It's crucial to be frank and honest while sharing your worries. Keep in mind that your medical professionals are there to assist you and have probably dealt with similar issues from other patients in the past. A more cooperative and sympathetic connection with your healthcare team can result from sharing your concerns.

Concerns can also be expressed through nonverbal clues in addition to vocal communication. Be aware of your body language because it frequently reveals feelings that are difficult to explain in words. Maintain eye contact, make welcoming gestures, and pay attention to your healthcare providers' nonverbal clues. This will promote an information exchange that is more honest and kind.

Active Participation in Decision-Making:

It's important for you to actively engage in making healthcare decisions if you have brittle bone disease. It is crucial to express your preferences and values in order to receive the most individualised care from your healthcare providers when they offer you with different treatment alternatives or management techniques.

To actively participate in decision-making, it is important to:

1. Be informed: Learn as much as you can about the various treatment options, including any potential advantages, hazards, and long-term effects. As a result, you'll be able to decide according to your own demands and ideals.

2. Prioritize your goals: When choosing a course of treatment, take your unique priorities and aspirations into account. To make sure the proposed treatment will lead to the results you want, talk about them with your healthcare professionals.

3. Voice your preferences: Tell the medical staff about your preferences. This may entail things like taking non-invasive treatment choices into account, reducing pharmaceutical side effects, or giving pain management top priority.

4. Seek a second opinion if necessary: Don't be afraid to get a second opinion if you have questions about a recommended treatment course of action or would like to consider other possibilities. You may gain more clarity and confidence in your decision-making as a result.

Always keep in mind that communication is two-way. You must actively listen while also clearly expressing your demands and concerns. You may guarantee that your voice is heard and valued in the treatment process by actively participating in your healthcare decisions.

Conclusion:

Receiving high-quality care for brittle bone disease depends on effective communication with medical professionals. You may speak out for your own needs, get individualised care, and have better health outcomes by voicing your concerns, asking questions, and actively engaging in the decision-making process. To ensure the greatest care for your illness, keep in mind to bring a list of questions, be honest and upfront about your worries, and actively participate with your healthcare team.

Collaborative Care and Treatment Planning

A team of professionals from several health and wellness sectors must collaborate when it comes to Brittle Bone Disease, commonly known as Osteogenesis Imperfecta. Because of this disease's effects on the bones, they become excessively brittle and prone to breaking. But other parts of the body are also impacted. This condition may also affect a person's overall health and well-being. Because of this, it's crucial to adopt a multidisciplinary strategy to guarantee a thorough and all-encompassing treatment strategy.

The capacity to handle all of the numerous facets of Brittle Bone Disease is one of the main advantages of interdisciplinary care. With a group of specialists, we may concentrate not only on a person's physical health but also on their mental and emotional well-being. This method acknowledges the connection between the physical and mental facets of health and the necessity of addressing both for the best results.

For instance, people with Brittle Bone Disease frequently experience persistent pain from fractures and other side effects. It is crucial to have pain management specialists in addition to orthopaedic doctors who can perform medical interventions because they can help reduce pain using a variety of methods, including medication, physical therapy, and alternative therapies. With a team of specialists, we can offer a thorough approach to pain treatment, treating the underlying reasons and striving to enhance the quality of life for the patient.

Involving the patient and their relatives in the decision-making process is also crucial. Through the use of shared decision-making, patients are given the ability to actively engage in their care, comprehend the options accessible to them, and make decisions that are tailored to their individual requirements and preferences. Goals, ideals, and aspirations of the individual must be taken into account.

By integrating the patient in the decision-making process, we boost not only their compliance and adherence to the plan but also their satisfaction with the therapy.

With a coordinated care strategy, the entire healthcare team is on the same page and working toward the same objectives. Effective communication, information sharing, and consistent follow-up are required. In the case of Brittle Bone Disease, when numerous specialists may be engaged in the patient's care, coordination is especially crucial. To maintain the best possible bone health, for instance, orthopaedic surgeons may need to work with endocrinologists. To increase mobility and improve everyday functioning, physical therapists and occupational therapists may collaborate together. We can make sure the person receives smooth and integrated care by encouraging collaboration and communication across the various providers.

In my clinical experience, I have observed how coordinated care and treatment planning benefit patients with Brittle Bone Disease. We can create a thorough and tailored treatment plan that covers every aspect of the problem by bringing together experts from various professions. This method boosts the person's general wellbeing and quality of life in addition to their physical health.

Let me use the example of one of my patients, Lisa, to highlight the value of collaborative treatment. Lisa, a young adult in her twenties, has had brittle bone disease since she was a child. She has had multiple fractures and frequently felt helpless and irritated when trying to control her condition. She was overwhelmed and unsure of her treatment options when she initially came to see me.

We began by putting together a group of professionals, which included psychiatrists, physical therapists, pain management experts, and orthopaedic surgeons. With regard to various facets of Lisa's health, each provider was vital to her care. The orthopaedic specialists concentrated on treating her fractures and making sure that her bones were properly aligned. She was able to move more freely and build strength thanks to the physical therapists. Her persistent pain was reduced by the pain management professionals with the use of a combination of prescription drugs and complementary treatments. The psychologists assisted Lisa in addressing her mental issues and gave her coping mechanisms for dealing with the difficulties of having brittle bone disease.

Lisa fully engaged in the creation of her treatment plan through collaborative decision-making. She indicated a desire for a more autonomous lifestyle and to pursue her professional ambitions. In light of this, we created a treatment strategy for her that included controlling her fractures as well as enhancing her stamina and endurance. The length of Lisa's physical therapy sessions was increased, and she gradually began adding consistent exercise to her daily routine. In addition, we gave her the tools and encouragement she needed to look into medically accommodating job choices.

All members of the healthcare team were brought together through the coordinated care strategy, ensuring effective communication and follow-up. We were able to discuss Lisa's progress at regular team meetings, make any changes to Lisa's treatment plan, and deal with any issues or difficulties that emerged. Because of this coordination, Lisa received a holistic and integrated care experience. Rather than being fragmented, her treatment was made up of several puzzle pieces that fit together to provide a whole picture of her well-being.

Lisa's condition greatly improved over time. She suffered fewer fractures, improved at managing her pain, and had faith in her capacity to overcome the difficulties of brittle bone disease and lead a happy life. In addition to addressing the medical components of her condition, the collaborative care model gave her the support and resources she needed to deal with the disease's emotional and psychological effects.

In conclusion, managing Brittle Bone Disease requires coordinated care and treatment planning. Given the complexity of this condition, an interdisciplinary approach, collaborative decision-making, and coordinated care are crucial. We can offer people a thorough and holistic treatment plan that focuses not only on their physical health but also on their mental and emotional well-being by bringing together professionals from several health and wellness sectors. Through cooperation, we can enable people to take an active role in their care, enhance their general quality of life, and ease their path to optimum health and wellness..

Advocating for Comprehensive Care

Ensuring Access to Necessary Services:

Accessing the services required for their care is one of the biggest obstacles people with Brittle Bone Disease confront. The availability of specialised medical personnel and facilities may be constrained due to the condition's rarity. Financial limitations and insurance coverage might also restrict the types of care that are available.

It is essential to establish a strong network of relationships and resources in order to get over these obstacles. As a doctor, I have made it a point to develop connections with other medical experts that focus on treating Brittle Bone Disease. I am able to offer my patients a thorough and multidisciplinary approach to their care by working with specialists in orthopaedics, genetics, and physical therapy.

In addition to creating a network of medical experts, advocating at the structural and organisational levels is crucial. We can collectively campaign for more funding for research into brittle bone disease and the establishment of specialist treatment facilities by collaborating with patient advocacy groups and professional associations. These facilities can thus act as focal points for comprehensive care, guaranteeing that those who have the condition can receive all necessary services in a single location..

Coordinating Care:

The efficient coordination of a patient's medical care is a crucial component of providing complete care for those with Brittle Bone Disease. It is my duty as the patient's primary care physician to function as the patient's main point of contact and to coordinate the efforts of the numerous specialists involved in their treatment.

I use a team-based strategy to do this, including experts from several health and wellness disciplines. Orthopedists, genetic counsellors, physical therapists, dietitians, and psychologists are some of the members of this team. We are able to create individualised treatment regimens that take into account each person's particular needs by cooperating.

All members of the healthcare team must communicate clearly and openly in order for care coordination to be effective. To make sure that everyone is in agreement with the patient's development and treatment objectives, regular meetings and case conferences are helpful. The patient and their family are included as active participants in their care as part of this coordination, which goes beyond the healthcare team. We enable them to take an active role in controlling their condition by including them in the decision-making process, educating them, and offering them support.

Addressing Healthcare Disparities:

Healthcare inequities do, unfortunately, exist, even in the case of brittle bone disease. Disparities in access to care, the standard of care received, and health outcomes are just a few ways in which these disparities might appear. As a supporter of holistic healthcare, I'm dedicated to tackling these inequities and making sure that everyone with brittle bone disease has fair access to complete care.

To do this, it is crucial to have a thorough grasp of the distinctive difficulties that various communities impacted by Brittle Bone Disease experience. People from underprivileged populations, for instance, may encounter additional obstacles including prejudice, restricted access to transportation, or language challenges. We may try to reduce inequities and improve health outcomes by proactively addressing these factors and provide culturally competent treatment.

In order to recognise and treat healthcare disparities, research and data collecting are also vital. We can pinpoint areas for improvement and push for systemic policy changes by actively participating in research activities and gathering data on the experiences and outcomes of people with Brittle Bone Disease.

In the end, promoting comprehensive care necessitates a wholistic and patient-centered strategy. We can give people with Brittle Bone

Disease the best care and assistance by guaranteeing access to essential services, coordinating care, and eliminating healthcare disparities. I'm committed to continue to speak out for and provide complete care for these people as a medical professional and health and wellness coach, making sure they have the tools and encouragement they need to lead full and satisfying lives.

Navigating the Healthcare System

Insurance Coverage:

Knowing your insurance coverage is one of the first and most crucial things to keep in mind when navigating the healthcare system. It's crucial to study your policy and comprehend what is covered and what is not because insurance companies have varying policies when it comes to coverage for Brittle Bone Disease.

I advise getting in touch with your insurance company first and asking for a thorough breakdown of your coverage. This will make it easier for you to comprehend your policy's particular terms and conditions, including any restrictions or Brittle Bone Disease exclusions. Additionally, it's crucial to maintain a record of any correspondence with your insurance provider, including conversations, emails, and letters. Should a dispute emerge in the future, this will show that you tried to understand your coverage.

Working with a healthcare advocate who focuses on insurance coverage for chronic diseases may also be helpful. These experts can assist you in navigating the frequently confusing insurance landscape and guarantee that you are making the most of your Brittle Bone Disease coverage. They can also help you get the appropriate treatments and medications and appeal any claims that have been rejected.

Medical Records Management:

Managing your medical data efficiently is a crucial part of navigating the healthcare system. In addition to recording your medical history, medical records are essential for brittle bone disease diagnosis, management, and treatment.

Gathering and organising all of your medical documents pertaining to brittle bone disease is crucial. This covers test outcomes, physician notes, treatment schedules, and any other pertinent paperwork. Make copies of these documents for backup purposes, and keep them in a secure location that is easy to access.

Next, think about adopting a healthcare app or a personal health record (PHR) to keep track of your medical data. By using these technologies, you may update and keep your records digitally, making them readily available anytime you need them. You may even be able to share your records with your healthcare professionals through some PHRs, providing continuity of care and lowering the possibility that any details will be missing or ignored.

Maximizing Healthcare Resources:

It's critical to make the most of the healthcare services at your disposal in addition to comprehending your insurance coverage and managing your medical records. In order to effectively manage your disease, you will need a multidisciplinary approach to care from a variety of clinicians and agencies.

First off, I urge you to choose a specialist medical team that consists of experts in domains like orthopaedics, physical therapy, nutrition, and mental health. A thorough and individualised treatment and care plan will be created by this team for your brittle bone disease. You will receive a wide range of lifestyle adjustments, dietary guidance, counseling- and psychology-related approaches, alternative and complementary self-care methods, self-help methods, and coping mechanisms from them.

It's also critical to keep up with new developments and research in the field of brittle bone disease. Join support groups, go to conferences or webinars, and follow trustworthy businesses and subject-matter authorities. This will not only keep you informed but also provide you access to a network of people who can assist and direct you as you travel.

Finally, don't be afraid to get in touch with patient advocacy groups that focus on brittle bone disease. These groups are committed to helping those who have the illness and can offer useful tools, knowledge, and support. They might also be able to put you in touch with people or families who are also struggling with brittle bone disease so you can exchange knowledge, counsel, and emotional support.

In conclusion, navigating the healthcare system might be difficult, but you can successfully treat your Brittle Bone Disease with the appropriate approaches. Spend some time learning about your insurance coverage, managing and organising your medical information, and making the most of the tools at your disposal. Do not forget that you are not alone in this path; seek out help from healthcare advocates, specialist healthcare teams, patient advocacy groups, and networks. Adopting this interdisciplinary and holistic approach will provide you the tools you need to manage your health and lead a happy, full life.

Chapter 12: Empowering the Brittle Bone Disease Community

Creating Supportive Networks and Organizations

For people with Brittle Bone Disease and their loved ones who might also need help and understanding, support groups can be a lifeline. People who are struggling with similar issues can gather in these groups, discuss their experiences, and offer support to one another. They act as a safe haven. It is critical to realise that support groups can be set up in a variety of ways, based on community preferences and needs. They might be physical gatherings held at neighbourhood community centres, medical facilities, or clinics, or they can be online communities run through tools like social media forums or video conferencing software.

Here are some ideas to get you going if you want to organise a support group for people with brittle bone disease:

1. Identify the Need: Consider the demand and interest within the Brittle Bone Disease community before jumping into the creation of a support group. Connect with those who are impacted by the condition, find out their ideas and preferences, and gauge their level of interest in joining a group like this.

2. Establish Goals and Objectives: Define your support group's aims and objectives after determining the necessity. Are you hoping to coordinate social activities, share resources and information, or offer emotional support? Make sure your goal is clear and in line with the community's requirements.

3. Recruit Members: Share information about your support group with local medical facilities, clinics, community centres, and websites for people with rare diseases. Encourage Brittle Bone Disease sufferers and their families to join the organisation and take an active role in it.

4. Organize Meetings: Determine the meeting schedule and format for your support group. If you're organising meetings in person,

find a good location that is also accessible to people with physical limitations. Choose a reputable platform that enables simple communication and involvement for virtual meetings.

5. Facilitate Discussions: As a facilitator, it's critical to establish a welcoming environment where people feel free to freely express their ideas, worries, and experiences. Organize your meetings to include both educational presentations and free-flowing discussions so that attendees may interact.

6. Provide Resources: Consider establishing a list of pertinent resources, such as financial assistance programmes, adaptive equipment suppliers, and medical practitioners that specialise in Brittle Bone Disease. Members of your support group should be informed about these resources on a regular basis.

Online networks are essential for bringing people with Brittle Bone Disease together across geographical borders, in addition to support groups. Creating an online platform, such as a social media page or specific website, gives people a place to go for support, inspiration, and knowledge whenever they want. Online networks also foster a sense of community and lessen the isolation that frequently comes with uncommon diseases.

Similar steps are involved in starting an online community for Brittle Bone Disease as in starting a support group. There are a few other things to bear in mind, though:

1. Choose an Appropriate Platform: Choose an appropriate internet platform that can meet your community's demands. Make sure the platform you select enables simple communication, content sharing, and privacy settings to safeguard the members' identities and personal data.

2. Promote Active Participation: Encourage participants to actively participate in the community by talking about their experiences, asking for help, and supporting their neighbours. Facilitate conversations and

develop chances for people to develop closer relationships with one another.

3. Provide Reliable Information: It is crucial to make sure that the data given on the platform is accurate and trustworthy as a community organiser. Encourage members to seek counsel from reputable healthcare specialists rather than endorsing unsupported claims or therapies.

Supporting the needs of the community and promoting improved treatment are all important goals of advocacy groups for Brittle Bone Disease. These groups frequently engage in a range of activities, including raising money for research, running awareness campaigns, and promoting legislation that will help those who are afflicted by the condition.

Here are a few things to think about if you want to start an advocacy group for people with brittle bone disease and are passionate about doing so:

1. Define Your Purpose: Clearly state your organization's goals and objectives. Decide if you want to concentrate on promoting awareness, funding research, promoting policies, or a combination of these objectives.

2. Form a Team: Speak to others who are as passionate as you are about helping people with brittle bone disease. Assemble a group of people with similar viewpoints who can provide their knowledge and abilities to the organization's efforts.

3. Register Your Organization: You might need to register your advocacy organisation as a nonprofit or charity entity, depending on the laws in your nation. To guarantee compliance with all necessary regulations, seek legal counsel.

4. Establish Partnerships: To increase the impact of your organization's actions, work with medical personnel, healthcare facilities, research organisations, and other advocacy groups.

Partnerships can help you reach a wider audience and provide you access to more resources.

5. Plan Fundraising Activities: Find prospective sources of funding for the objectives and projects of your organisation. This may entail pursuing grants, planning fund-raising activities, developing online donation systems, or forming alliances with commercial sponsors.

6. Advocate for Change: Engage with decision-makers, governing bodies, and medical institutions to promote laws and programmes that enhance the quality of life for those who suffer from brittle bone disease. Support research initiatives and use a variety of platforms to spread awareness of the issue.

In order to guarantee that those with the condition and their families receive the assistance, tools, and empowerment they require, supportive networks and organisations for the community of people with brittle bone disease must be established. We can all work together to create support groups, online communities, and advocacy organisations to improve the quality of life for those with this rare condition. Keep in mind that when we work together, we are stronger and can achieve more.

Raising Awareness and Challenging Stigma

Raising awareness of the condition itself is important in addressing the stigma connected to brittle bone disease. Because so few people are aware of or understand this uncommon genetic ailment, it can result in misunderstandings and prejudice against persons who have it. I feel it is my responsibility as a doctor and a health and wellness coach to inform the public and attempt to dispel these stereotypes.

It's critical to give accurate information on Brittle Bone Disease in order to properly increase awareness. Sharing information regarding the causes, symptoms, and possible treatments can fall under this category. It is essential to debunk any myths or false beliefs that might be spread by the media or the general public. We can contribute to a better knowledge of the ailment and lessen the stigma associated with it by disseminating factual information.

Advocacy is essential in battling stigma in addition to knowledge provision. It entails advocating for and standing by people who have brittle bone disease. Participating in awareness campaigns, planning public education events, and collaborating with legislators to ensure the needs of persons with the condition are met are just a few examples of the numerous ways advocacy can take place. We can build a more welcoming and compassionate society by fighting for the rights and welfare of these people.

Another effective approach for combating stigma is education. We can contribute to ensuring that persons suffering with Brittle Bone Disease receive the right support and treatment by educating healthcare workers, educators, and other important stakeholders. This may entail offering instruction on how to successfully manage and meet the requirements of those who have the condition. Public education may also entail using workshops, school programmes, and online resources. We can close the comprehension gap by educating people and giving them authority.

In order to change public perceptions of brittle bone disease, we must also confront our own prejudices and preconceptions. Humans have a propensity to fear the unknown, and this anxiety frequently results in stigmatisation and prejudice. We need to actively engage in self-reflection and face our own biases in order to get over this. We must understand that people with brittle bone disease are defined by their special skills, talents, and personalities rather than by their illness.

Supporting persons who have Brittle Bone Disease as well as their families is also crucial. Support groups and counselling programmes can be quite helpful in assisting people in overcoming the difficulties brought on by the condition. They can give a secure setting for exchanging stories, giving counsel, and building a sense of community. By introducing people to others who have gone through similar things, we can lessen their sense of loneliness and give them the tools they need to overcome any barriers they may encounter.

It's crucial to keep in mind that change takes time while working to eradicate the stigma attached to brittle bone disease. Individuals, healthcare professionals, advocacy organisations, and policymakers must all work together to achieve this. Together, we can build a society that is more accepting, sympathetic, and helpful to people with the disease.

In conclusion, improving the lives of people with Brittle Bone Disease requires increasing knowledge and dispelling the stigma attached to the condition. We can build a more kind and inclusive society by giving factual information, standing up for their needs, and educating the general public. We must confront our prejudices and encourage those who have Brittle Bone Disease by giving them the tools and chances they require to prosper. Together, we can remove obstacles and build a society that values and respects people with brittle bone disease.

Sharing Resources and Information

The sharing of information and support within the healthcare industry has become one of my most valuable insights throughout the years. I have seen personally the advantages of sharing resources and information, particularly when it comes to rare conditions like Brittle Bone Disease. I am a doctor and a health and wellness coach.

Coming together as a community has tremendous power, and this is especially true in the case of brittle bone disease. By exchanging tools and knowledge, we may not only inform ourselves and others about the situation, but also give people the power to take charge of their own health and wellbeing.

The internet is one of the most important resources in the current day. Online tools have completely changed how we communicate, share, and learn. There are a number of online sites that can be a great resource for information and support for people who have brittle bone disease.

The Brittle Bone Society website is one such resource. It offers a plethora of information on the ailment, as well as the most recent studies, treatment choices, and support services. Additionally, it provides a forum where people may interact with others who have the illness, exchange stories, and get support.

Social media is a further online resource that shouldn't be disregarded. Social media sites like Facebook, Instagram, and Twitter have developed into effective tools for bringing individuals from different backgrounds together. People can interact with people who have the same illness and learn more about their experiences and coping mechanisms by joining groups dedicated to Brittle Bone Disease and by following hashtags that are pertinent to the condition.

It is essential to look into educational resources that offer in-depth knowledge about Brittle Bone Disease in addition to online resources. One such tool is the book "Brittle Bone Disease: A Comprehensive

Guide," which was written by renowned expert Dr. Sarah Thompson. This in-depth manual explores the many forms of brittle bone disease, diagnostic techniques, available treatments, and management techniques.

Additionally, there are a tonne of academic publications and studies that discuss the different facets of brittle bone disease. The biomedical literature database PubMed is a great place to find these investigations. People can stay up to date on the most recent breakthroughs and discoveries in the industry by staying current with the research.

Another effective method of sharing resources and knowledge within the community affected by Brittle Bone Disease is through collaborative efforts. In order to work collaboratively on research, treatment paradigms, and patient care, these initiatives bring together professionals from many health and wellness sectors. One such instance is the Brittle Bone Disease Research Consortium, which brings together researchers, doctors, and patient advocates to advance knowledge of the disorder and enhance patient outcomes.

In addition to working together professionally, fostering a sense of community among people with Brittle Bone Disease is crucial. This can be accomplished through online and offline support groups, where people can interact with others who genuinely comprehend their struggles and victories. An excellent illustration of one of these initiatives is the local hospital's Brittle Bone Disease Support Group. People can talk about their experiences, give each other advice, and get emotional support in these support groups.

Within the network for people with brittle bone disease, anyone can share materials and knowledge. People can actively participate in this process by sharing their own experiences, perceptions, and coping mechanisms. You can do this by writing on personal blogs, posting on social media, or taking part in patient-led initiatives.

People can provide others suffering comparable difficulties hope, motivation, and useful advice by sharing their own personal tales and experiences. Being reminded that they are not alone in their path and that there are ways to live happy lives despite the restrictions imposed by Brittle Bone Disease, people can feel enormously empowered by this interchange of information and support.

The importance of sharing resources and knowledge within the Brittle Bone Disease community cannot be overstated, in conclusion. Individuals can better manage their health and well-being with the use of online platforms, educational resources, and cooperative projects, among other things. We can build a welcoming environment that encourages comprehension, resiliency, and optimism within the Brittle Bone Disease community by combining our expertise, experiences, and resources..

Supporting Research and Fundraising

Participating in Clinical Trials:

Clinical trials are research projects that test new medicines for safety and efficacy on human subjects. They are essential to the development of medical knowledge and the enhancement of patient care. Clinical trial participation can provide people with Brittle Bone Disease hope for new therapies and potential breakthroughs.

Prior to enrolling in a clinical trial, it is crucial to conduct careful research and speak with medical experts. Start by looking for clinical trials that are especially geared toward the condition of brittle bones. Trial tools and information can be found on websites like clinicaltrials.gov and the Brittle Bone Society.

Once you have located a clinical trial that might be appropriate for you or a loved one, spend some time reading and comprehending the study's objectives, eligibility requirements, and any dangers. Understanding the trial's requirements and what is expected of participants is essential.

If you choose to take part, get in touch with the principle investigator or study organiser to let them know you're interested. They will walk you through the enrolling process and give you any information you require regarding the trial.

Being a part of a clinical study gives you access to cutting-edge medical procedures and specialised care in addition to helping progress science. Additionally, by opening the way for better therapies and new treatments, your involvement may help future generations affected by brittle bone disease.

Organizing Fundraisers:

In order to support research projects and spread awareness about Brittle Bone Disease, fundraising is essential. By working together to plan fundraisers, people and communities open up possibilities for having a real effect and advancing science.

A clear aim and strategy must be in place before planning a fundraising. Start by deciding whether the fundraiser's goal is to support those who are suffering from the ailment, generate money for research, or both. This will direct your decision-making and assist you in developing sound strategies.

Consider planning a range of events to involve various community groups. Physical wellbeing can be promoted while collecting money and awareness through fundraising walks, runs, or bike rides. Events like bake sales, benefit concerts, and charity auctions let people show off their skills while supporting a good cause. Partnerships with neighbourhood companies or organisations can also encourage a greater level of support and participation.

Be sure to consult relevant stakeholders, such as medical experts, researchers, and people with Brittle Bone Disease, in the design of your fundraising. Their knowledge and first-hand experience will offer priceless insights and ensure that your efforts are in line with community demands.

Don't forget to advertise your fundraiser using a variety of platforms, including social media, regional newspapers, and neighbourhood bulletin boards. Use social media to spread the word, and encourage friends, family, and coworkers to do the same. Additionally, requesting coverage from regional media channels might help your cause gain more recognition and support.

Contributing to Scientific Advancements:

There are additional ways people can help progress science in the area of brittle bone disease besides taking part in clinical studies and planning fundraisers. Giving to organisations and foundations that specialise in research and support for this condition is a powerful way to make a difference.

There are numerous organisations, like the Brittle Bone Society, whose main goals are to enhance research, offer assistance to those who are affected and their families, and promote better healthcare laws. You can directly support these organisations' work by making a donation. These contributions support research projects, offer resources to patients, and increase public awareness of the illness.

Additionally, it's important to keep up with the most recent discoveries and developments in the science of brittle bone disease. Read scholarly publications, go to seminars and conferences, and communicate with medical experts and researchers via social media and online discussion boards. This information will assist you in staying informed and choosing the best therapies and sources of support for you or your loved ones.

Participating actively in patient registries and studies looking into brittle bone disease is another opportunity to give back. These programmes gather important information that may help us understand the problem better and develop treatments and cures. You actively participate in the research process and advance the field of science by contributing your experiences and insights.

In conclusion, it is critical to fund research into Brittle Bone Disease in order to advance medical knowledge, enhance patient care, and perhaps even discover a solution. People may significantly improve the lives of those affected by this ailment by taking part in clinical studies, planning fundraisers, and advancing science. Together, we can create a future in which Brittle Bone Disease is a controllable and treatable condition rather than a cause for worry and uncertainty..

Inspiring Hope and Celebrating Strength

It is without a doubt difficult to live with brittle bone disease on both an emotional and physical level. But it's critical to keep in mind that there is always cause for optimism and that courage may be discovered in the most unlikely of places. I've spent years dealing with patients, and during that time I've seen innumerable examples of people who have not only managed to flourish in spite of their illness, but who have also turned into lights of hope and inspiration for those going through similar difficulties.

One of these triumph stories is Sarah, a young person who has battled brittle bone disease her entire life. After learning of her diagnosis, Sarah was immediately saddened and despondent. Nevertheless, she made a conscious choice to take control of her life and look for methods to recognise her power rather than letting negativity to overtake her. Sarah developed a love for art through her experience and started utilising her skill to both express herself and spread awareness of brittle bone disease. Her work has impacted the lives of numerous others, inspiring hope, and eradicating the stigma attached to the condition. She now has a thriving profession as an artist.

The Brittle Bone Disease community's tenacity and tenacity are demonstrated by Sarah's tale, which is only one of many. The incident is not unique, though. Many people have been able to find meaning and purpose in their life in addition to overcoming the physical obstacles presented by the condition. These triumphs serve as a reminder that, even though Brittle Bone Disease may present its own set of challenges, it does not define who we are or what we are capable of.

Recognizing the strength that comes from a group of people working together is also crucial. The close-knit community for those with brittle bone disease gives its members unwavering support and inspiration. People can find others who actually understand their challenges and connect with them through support groups, online forums, and social media platforms. They can also share experiences, offer guidance, and offer words of encouragement. This sense of belonging and community serves as a source of inspiration and fortitude in addition to fostering a sense of belonging.

Additionally, studies have demonstrated that people who take an active role in community involvement and support organisations benefit mentally and generally from their lives. People with brittle bone disease may feel less alone as a result of their sense of connection and belonging, which gives them the confidence to take on the challenges of the condition. By highlighting the community's strengths, we not only encourage one another but also instil confidence in the next generation.

Along with the help of the neighbourhood, adopting a holistic approach to heath and wellbeing is essential for fostering optimism and honouring strength. We believe in offering our patients comprehensive care at my clinic, which extends beyond merely offering medical care. We are aware of how crucial it is to take into account the social, emotional, and psychological effects of having brittle bone disease. This entails empowering people through lifestyle adjustments, food and diet planning, counselling and psychology-related procedures, various self-care alternatives and complementary techniques, self-help tactics, and coping mechanisms.

We are able to offer a comprehensive framework that encourages resiliency, hope, and strength by taking into account all facets of a person's wellbeing. Our patients are urged to pursue their interests, derive significance from their life experiences, and appreciate their own journeys. Using individualised care plans, we assist people in creating coping strategies, a solid network of allies, and a positive outlook.

The importance of advocacy should be highlighted last. We may dismantle obstacles and foster an atmosphere that promotes strength and resiliency by educating the general public about Brittle Bone

Disease and its difficulties and successes. We can encourage inclusivity and give people with Brittle Bone Disease the tools they need to live life to the fullest by launching public campaigns, launching educational programmes, and showcasing them in the media.

The community for people with brittle bone disease is incredibly strong, and we can celebrate this by sharing success stories, displaying resiliency, and emphasising the power of people working together. We can foster an environment in which people with Brittle Bone Disease can thrive, find meaning, and motivate others through a holistic approach to healthcare and wellbeing, community support, and activism. While the path may be difficult, let's not forget that there is always hope and strength available to us.

www.ingramcontent.com/pod-product-compliance
Lightning Source LLC
LaVergne TN
LVHW011756150625
813908LV00012B/714